Moody, Jane

Breastfeeding your baby

Breastfeeding Your Baby

Jane Moody, Jane Britten and Karen Hogg

A
NATIONAL CHILDBIRTH TRUST
GUIDE

Published by National Childbirth Trust Publishing
in collaboration with Thorsons

Thorsons
An Imprint of HarperCollins*Publishers*

NCT
EDITIONS

Picture Acknowledgements

The publishers would like to thank the following for their permission to
reproduce photographs: Camilla Jessel: Cover; Joanne O'Brien: pxiv;
The National Childbirth Trust: pp20, 42, 58, 146; Michael Bassett: pp86, 98, 208;
David Muscroft: p110; Julian Cotton Photo Library: pp128, 162; Egnell Ameda: p188.

Illustrations: Mike Edwards, Pete Welford,
Jo Dennis.

Design by Tim McPhee.

Production in association with
Book Production Consultants plc,
25-27 High Street, Chesterton, Cambridge CB4 1ND, UK.

Printed by Hillman Printers (Frome) Ltd,
Frome, Somerset.

Published by National Childbirth Trust Publishing,
25-27 High Street, Chesterton, Cambridge CB4 1ND, UK.

in collaboration with Thorsons
An Imprint of HarperCollins *Publishers*
77–85 Fulham Palace Road, Hammersmith, London W6 8JB.

© 1996 NCT Publishing

First published 1996
This edition 1998

A CIP catalogue record for this book is available from the British Library.

ISBN 0 7225 3635 6

Contents

About the authors

Jane Britten has had a great interest in breastfeeding since the birth of her first son in 1985. She is a breastfeeding counsellor and is breastfeeding editor of *New Generation*, the journal of the NCT. She is currently co-ordinating an infant feeding audit in Glasgow, where she lives.

Jane Moody has been involved with the NCT since 1981. She is a breastfeeding counsellor and tutor for the Trust and edits the *New Generation Digest*. She also works as a freelance copy-editor and occasional journalist.

Karen Hogg has been involved with the NCT since 1979. She is a breastfeeding counsellor and tutor for the Trust, and works as a freelance lecturer and professional counsellor.

Publisher's note

ALL COMMENTS and personal accounts were given to us in confidence, so out of respect for our contributors' privacy we have changed all the names.

We have endeavoured where possible to reproduce quotations verbatim, but where editing has been applied, the integrity of the quotation has been maintained.

Acknowledgements

FIRSTLY, AND most importantly, thank you to all the mothers who wrote about their personal experiences of breastfeeding, for their courage in telling us their stories, even when it was painful to do so, and for their keenness to share their enjoyment of breastfeeding with other mothers. This book would not exist without them.

We owe a huge debt of thanks to our families, who encouraged us in this project. In particular, our husbands, who helped when word processors refused to co-operate and listened when we needed them.

Thank you to Sally Inch for allowing us first use of her table; to Ruth Dumbreck for checking our information on the Baby Friendly Hospital Initiative; to Patricia Donnithorne, NCT Information Officer, for her swift and efficient response to pleas for photocopies and references; to Sheila Perkins for her very positive support; to Rayanne O'Neill and Connie for their 'First 14 days'; and to Rona McCandish and Mary Smale for reading the draft so diligently.

This book is dedicated to Stuart and Robbie Coleman; Adrienne, Matthew, Victoria and Philippa Hogg; Ruth and Thomas Moody – who began our interest in breastfeeding.

June 1995

Introduction

'Feeding my son has got to be one of my greatest achievements ever and the most fulfilling experience of my life.'

THIS BOOK began life as a leaflet and grew – the volume of information and personal stories grew so large that it could not possibly be contained in one leaflet. The leaflet was to be called *Women's Experiences of Breastfeeding*, and our book has taken that theme and expanded it. Nearly 200 women have contributed their personal experiences of breastfeeding, either for the original leaflet or specifically for our book. We owe them all a tremendous debt of gratitude for their frankness, their detailed responses and their enthusiasm for passing on their wisdom. 'Feeding Files' give you information to help you with the practicalities of breastfeeding, 'Background Notes' give you the facts.

We hope that the experiences of these women will give a picture of the real-life world of breastfeeding in the 1990s. We do not promise that it will all be easy if you read these pages; we do hope that if you are approaching becoming a parent, or if you are a breastfeeding mother, you will find someone here who echoes your thoughts and feelings. We do not aim to tell you 'how to do' breastfeeding, although we hope that you will find most of the information you need within these pages. We also hope that we have included helpful suggestions and background information to help you to make your own choices.

This is an exciting time for breastfeeding. Many hospitals are taking up the challenge of becoming Baby Friendly, and many more are realising that, up to now, there has been a gap between saying that breastfeeding is best – for you and for your baby – and providing good quality practical help and positive support and encouragement once your baby is born. It is into this gap that many mothers have fallen in the past. They know that they want to breastfeed, and often have a very detailed knowledge of how it should work. However, they have found that this has not been enough to enable them to succeed.

Our book follows your experience of breastfeeding through from your first memories and views about breastfeeding, through your experiences as a first-time mother – in hospital and at home – to your growing confidence as a breastfeeding mother. We look at introducing other foods to your baby and consider some views on how long breastfeeding should last. We take you through thinking about another baby and how to manage breastfeeding a baby while coping with a toddler, and what your experience might be if you are expecting twins. We look in some detail at various problems and difficulties which you might come across, and offer helpful information and suggestions for coping with and overcoming them, without giving up breastfeeding. We also look at some special experiences for both mother and baby. We explore the considerations around going back to work and continuing breastfeeding; and finally look at issues involved in stopping breastfeeding.

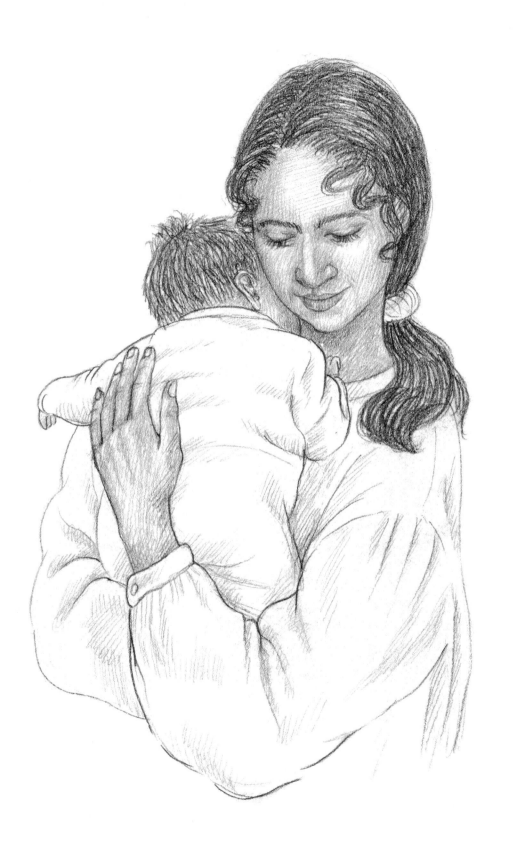

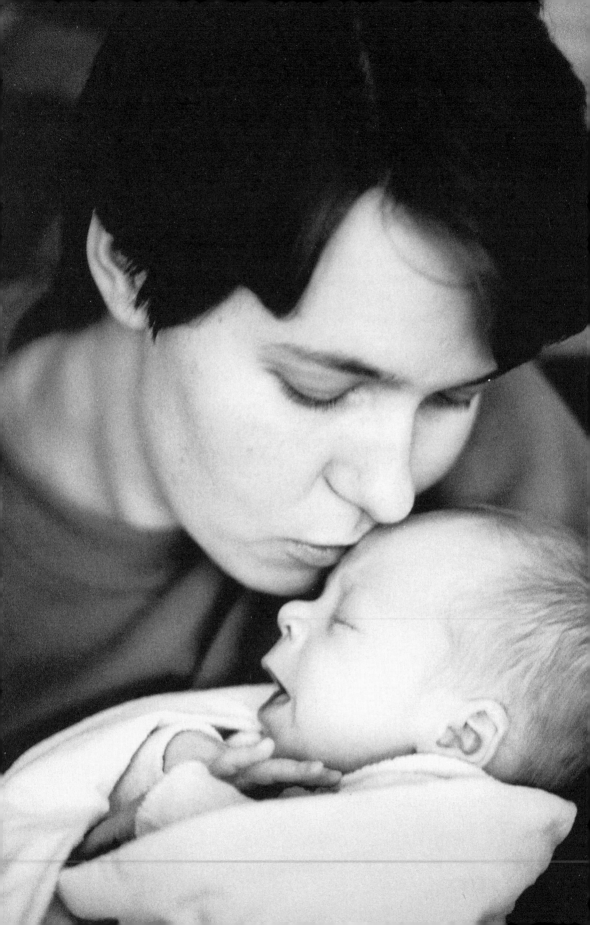

CHAPTER **_one_** *Before*
you begin

BREASTFEEDING IS an emotive subject: it is hard not to react when you hear the word. It involves a strong emotional response, from the mother who may be pregnant and thinking about feeding her baby; from the midwives and doctors who are caring for her, who may have personal experiences which colour their responses; from the woman's family, who may have equally strong views.

Our response is conditioned by our culture – in Western society, breasts mean sex, not baby feeding. This confusion of roles leads to much anxiety and uncertainty for some women, and definite rejection for others. By the time they are pregnant, most women have decided whether or not to breastfeed, even if they have not consciously thought about it.[1]

FIRST THOUGHTS OF BREASTFEEDING

BREASTFEEDING IS almost a lost art. Today, most of us have memories of seeing babies feeding from a bottle. The images come from everywhere: television, newspapers, even children's dolls often come with a feeding bottle full of 'milk' – tip the bottle up and the 'milk' disappears. It is hard to avoid the bottle-feeding culture. Breastfeeding has become something which is talked about, sometimes, but less often seen. Memories of breastfeeding seen in childhood are scarce. The images which remain are often vivid, though, as Clare explains: *'My own experiences of breastfeeding were very limited until I reached childbearing age. Most people I spoke to had tried to breastfeed and had not succeeded due to "pain" and "lack of milk" or "milk not strong enough". My mother had tried to breastfeed me, but in the sixties she was discouraged by the midwife and told, "modern women don't need to put up with all that". It was only my grandmother, who had breastfed three children during the War, who had the foresight to believe that women would once again realise the many benefits of breastfeeding.'*

Patricia stuck firmly to her earliest impressions of how breastfeeding would be: *'I remember hearing conversations about bottle-feeding: how convenient it was, how "civilised" and simple, but I always thought I'd breastfeed my children. I didn't want to share the feeding with anyone; I suppose as a child I had a very idealised picture of having a baby – just sitting down all day cuddling!'*

Ellen's first conscious memory of breastfeeding was when she was 12 or so: *'A young family friend, Sally, was breastfeeding her daughter and I seem to recall it was a bit of a talking point. I think there were mixed opinions about it. Some people were positively pleased to see a young mother succeed with breastfeeding, and some probably thought it was a bit weird, a bit hippie-ish for a conservative Australian rural area. It's odd how attitudes go round in circles! How natural breastfeeding can be seen as a bit weird and artificial feeding seen as the norm. I spent quite a bit of time with the family, babysitting and so on, and my younger sister is also a successful breastfeeder and supporter, so perhaps Sally deserves thanks for setting a good example.'*

WHERE A WOMAN has seen a mother breastfeeding her baby, the picture often remains with her and can affect how she feels about feeding her own babies.

Felicity's earliest memory of seeing a mother breastfeed her baby was a particularly peaceful one. When aged about 13, she went on a country ramble with her local youth group: *'One of the leaders had recently had a baby and when we stopped for a break she settled herself under a nearby tree, slightly away from the bustle of the energetic teenagers and calmly breastfed her baby. It was a beautiful scene with the sun filtering down through the leaves and I remember being quite fascinated by the mother and baby at peace with one another despite the noise and excitement around them. Although I don't recall thinking at the time, "when I have children I will breastfeed them", I believe the situation must have had some positive influence on me as I can clearly remember it nearly 20 years on.'*

Mothers can be very influential in forming a woman's attitude to breastfeeding. If a woman was herself breastfed, she is more likely to breastfeed her own children,[1] as Jennifer affirms: *'Before I had Richard, I had no doubt about breastfeeding. It was the only thing to do. I never considered bottle-feeding as an option. This was probably due to the recollection of a discussion years ago with my mum. I can't even remember how it came up but I remember her telling me all three of us were breastfed and she was very proud of it as a lot of mums had "stuck their babies on the bottle and that's why there are so many fat kids around now". I'm not sure where she got the evidence for the latter part of her statement but it left me with a lasting impression that breast milk was IT.'*

Elaine remembers her mum feeding her younger brother: *'I was nearly three at the time – she fed Mark for about a year. I also remember my mum's Dutch friend breastfeeding her baby, which was when I was seven. I was intrigued and felt comfortable sitting with them. Breastfeeding seemed the most natural thing for her to be doing. When I was ten, my mum had my younger sister . . . and she breastfed Amy for 18 months. I used to fetch and carry for her!'*

For Jane, a midwife, memories of baby feeding in her working environment are strong. The practices she describes are fairly typical of the 1970s, and it is not unknown to find 'hangovers' from this strict regime in some of today's hospitals: *'I worked on two wards where scheduled feeding was the rule. Feeding was four-hourly for two to three minutes each side increasing daily – no feeding at all for the first six hours except dextrose. I didn't realise how strange this was, but I can't remember being concerned about babies crying – and there were plenty of other things that horrified me. At night, the babies were all kept in the nursery and fed on evaporated milk – even when asked expressly not to – the mums just weren't told about it. It used to be called "white dextrose"!*

My lasting memory of the babies was how sleepy and "good" they were. We woke them up four hours after the start of their last feed, changed their nappies, gave them a bottle (most were bottle-fed). If they weren't drinking fast enough, the hole was enlarged. The feed had to be finished within 20 minutes – nappy changing took ten minutes and the babies were put back in their cots to sleep until their next feed. It all seemed so ordered and simple – how great was the contrast when Katy was born!

Just before Katy was born, it was recommended I read Breast Is Best *by P & A Stanway. It seems strange to think it now, but the book was revolutionary to me then. It was so positive and encouraging, breastfeeding became much more complex and interesting. The idea of demand feeding, mother and baby communicating, just the idea that your baby can be able and allowed to set the pace for feeding was completely new. In contrast with some hospitals where the baby is treated as the "enemy" to be forced to conform to a set of rules — to be allowed and encouraged to respond to my baby's needs as the Stanways suggested was wonderful.'*

DECIDING TO BREASTFEED

WOMEN GIVE many reasons for their decision to breastfeed. The most common are that breastfeeding is best for the baby, that it will be convenient and that it will lead to a closer bond between mother and baby.[1]

Emer was determined to breastfeed her first baby: *'With a history of asthma and eczema myself, having read around this subject, I knew my child would have a greater chance of not inheriting these problems if she was breastfed.'*

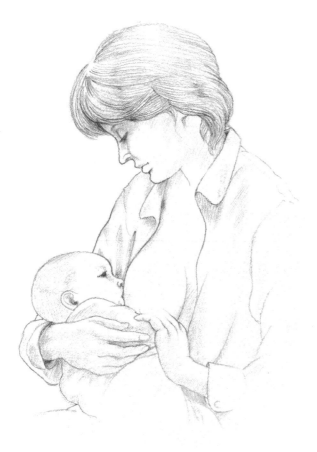

Amy recalls that the choice to breastfeed was made partly out of curiosity: *'I was aware that my brother and I had been bottle-fed. I also remember my aunt having her first child and being so ill with asthma after a caesarean that she was unable to breastfeed. She had wanted to, as she was taking the child back to live in Benghazi and knew that it was both cheaper and safer to breastfeed in that situation. Therefore I had only really seen women bottle-feeding although at the same time I was aware that breastfeeding was considered the best option. So when I came to have Timothy and was asked how I was going to feed, I chose to breastfeed without really having sought any support or information on the subject. I believed that all I had to do was choose.'*

BACKGROUND NOTES

Choices

In 1990, a survey was made of infant feeding in the United Kingdom.[1] Mothers were asked how they chose to feed their babies, and to give their reasons.

Choosing breastfeeding

● Breastfeeding is best for the baby. This reason was given by 82% of mothers
● Breastfeeding is more convenient – no bottles to prepare and no sterilising. 36% of mothers thought this important
● Bonding between mother and baby was thought to be better when the baby is breastfed by 23% of mothers
● Breastfeeding is cheaper than bottle-feeding. This was given as a reason for breastfeeding by 17% of mothers
● Among mothers who have breastfed a child, 29% gave their previous experience as a reason for breastfeeding again
● Breastfeeding is natural, felt by 14% to be important

● Breastfeeding is best for the mother too, and 8% of mothers gave this as a reason for breastfeeding
● Other reasons given by small numbers of women include the influence of health professionals and friends or relatives
● If a woman was herself breastfed, she is much more likely to want to breastfeed. 75% of women who were breastfed chose to breastfeed their own babies; 70% of women who were both breast and bottle-fed also chose breastfeeding, as did 48% of those who had been bottle-fed themselves
● If a mother's friends breastfeed, this is also an influence. 84% of women who said that most of their friends breastfed, planned to do the same.

Choosing bottle-feeding

● Other people can feed the baby. This was the most important reason for bottle-feeding for 39% of women
● Among mothers who had previously bottle-fed, 39% chose to do so again
● The idea of breastfeeding was not liked by 21% of mothers, and another 7% felt it was too embarrassing
● Seeing how much the baby has taken was felt to be a reason for choosing the bottle for 6% of mothers
● Medical reasons were given for bottle-feeding by 3% of mothers

● Returning to work soon after the birth was a reason for bottle-feeding for 5% of mothers
● Amongst other reasons given by small numbers of women, 1% reported having been persuaded to bottle-feed by other people
● If most of a mother's friends bottle-feed, 54% of women also choose to bottle-feed
● Mothers who were themselves bottle-fed are more likely to do the same: 52% of women who were bottle-fed planned to feed their baby this way.

BACKGROUND NOTES

What's special about breast milk?

Breast milk is a living fluid. It is made by you especially for your baby, so it is the most special food there is. No manufactured product can ever come close.

It is not possible to list all the ingredients in breast milk. Every new piece of research into this amazing fluid uncovers another vital ingredient which babies need for their development and growth.

Colostrum

Colostrum is extra special. It is rich in protein, immunoglobulins, vitamins, anti-infective agents, such as lactoferrin and lysozyme, living cells and minerals. Colostrum provides protection for the newborn baby until his own immune system begins to function, and ensures that his digestive system begins to function properly, as well as containing all the nutrients he needs.

The basic nutrients in breast milk

● Protein

Protein is needed for growth. Human babies are meant to grow slowly and feed often, so only a small proportion of human milk is protein: about 1%. Protein breaks down into curds (casein) and whey. Breast milk is largely whey, whereas cow's milk contains much more casein. Breast milk has no lactoglobulin, and it is thought that it is this part of the cow's milk protein, which is also present in infant formulas, which can cause allergic reactions.

● Carbohydrate

Nearly all of the carbohydrate in breast milk is lactose. It is important for brain growth, and the baby's brain is large and grows rapidly.

● Fat

Fat is needed to provide energy (calories). The fat in breast milk is very easily digested, with almost no waste. Essential long-chain fatty acids contained in breast milk have been found to be important for the growth and development of the baby's brain. These fatty acids are not naturally present in cow's milk or infant formula. Formula manufacturers are looking into the possibilities of including some of these fats in their products, but so far there is only one product available which includes any long-chain fatty acids.

● Water

Breast milk contains all the water a baby needs. Even in extreme heat or fever, a breastfed baby needs no extra water.

● Vitamins

Almost all women are able to provide all the vitamins for their baby's needs in their breast milk. A woman would have to be very obviously deficient in a vitamin for the levels in her breast milk to be less than adequate.

● Minerals

Although the iron content of breast milk is low, it is 20 times more easily absorbed than the iron in formula milk. Other minerals are present in ideal balances for the baby.

Added extras

This is where breast milk really scores over infant formula. Breast milk contains many 'non-nutritional' factors which help to protect and nurture the baby in his first few months: immunoglobulins, which help to protect the baby until his own immune system has developed; living cells, such as white cells for fighting infection; hormones and enzymes. All these add up to a truly unique substance which cannot be duplicated. Each mother produces the perfect food for *her* baby.

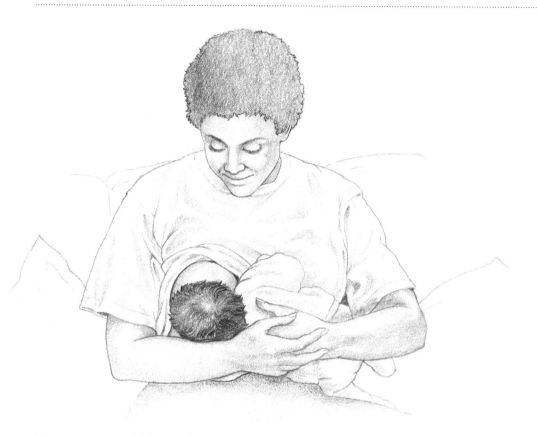

HOWEVER, THE feelings which underlie women's decisions to breast-feed are much more varied. Some women may feel anxious and lacking in confidence, which may be reinforced if their mothers or close friends did not breastfeed successfully. Others may be optimistic and self-assured, boosted by a supportive partner or friends with positive breastfeeding experiences. You may come to breastfeeding 'determined to succeed', or you may plan to 'give it a try and see what happens'. As Liz found, family influences are strong: *'Before my son was born I tried not to have any fixed ideas about anything I was going to do during or after the birth, but I was very keen to breastfeed my baby. I was a bit concerned as my mother had not been very successful at feeding either myself, my sister or my brother, but I was encouraged by my sister, who breastfed her son and then her daughter, born only six weeks before my son.'*

When Ruth trained as a nursery nurse, breastfeeding was very much promoted. However, her attitude became slightly coloured when she spent two weeks on a maternity ward: *'I was, for the first time, made*

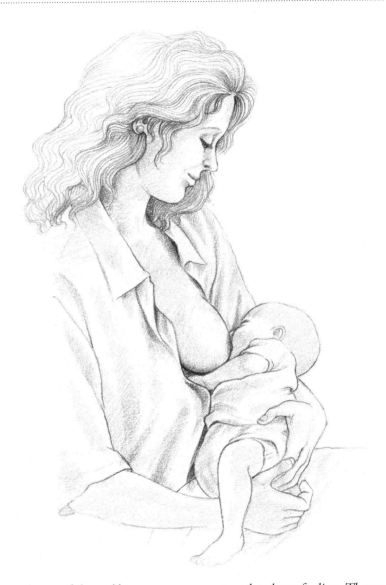

aware of some of the problems women encounter when breastfeeding. The vast majority of mothers were breastfeeding and although there were hints of a possible failure, my attitude was still "give it a good go", but for the first time, I felt that there could be problems.

After qualification I worked as a nanny. I found sterilising and making up bottles very tedious. The baby's feeding patterns were very varied, sometimes taking up to an hour to feed. These bottle-feeding experiences were actually quite valuable in reinforcing my inclination towards breastfeeding. I was sure bottle-feeding could be no easier or convenient than breast.'

PARTNERS CAN be very important: it is very hard for a woman to breastfeed if her partner does not support and encourage her. One study in America found that strong approval by the father of breast-feeding led to a high incidence of breastfeeding (98.1%), compared to only 26.9% when the father was indifferent to how his baby was fed.[2] Both Lois and her partner come from breastfeeding backgrounds. He was breastfed, as were his brother and sister, while her mother breast-fed all her four children: *'Soon after my husband and I discovered I was pregnant, we discussed how we would feed the baby and I was encouraged to hear that he was strongly in favour of my breastfeeding. This was a good ini-tial boost in that I then knew I could count on his whole-hearted support of my wish to breastfeed. I believe I would have been far less enthusiastic about breast-feeding had he been indifferent.'*

ALTHOUGH MANY women have already decided how they want to feed their baby before they become pregnant, the health professionals you meet during your pregnancy can have a profound influence on how you approach breastfeeding. Laura's experience was particularly disturbing: *'At an early antenatal appointment, a man in a white coat walked into the consulting room where the midwife was taking my blood pres-sure. He did not introduce himself, but I assume he was the consultant. He glanced at my notes, and asked me whether I intended to breastfeed. He squeezed my nipple really hard, grimaced and scribbled in his notes and walked out. I asked the midwife for an explanation and she said he probably thought that I would not be able to breastfeed as my nipples were very flat. When she saw my horrified expression she suggested that I start to pull my nipples out and roll them about in my fingers when having a bath. I couldn't believe I was hearing this, but left feeling depressed at the possibility of not being able to breastfeed and brought the subject up with my practice midwife. On examination, she said that she didn't think that it was a problem that a hungry baby couldn't sort out.'*

LEARNING ABOUT BREASTFEEDING

LEARNING ABOUT breastfeeding – both the theory and the practice – before the birth can be a way of boosting confidence. Antenatal classes run by the National Childbirth Trust usually include at least one session exclusively about breastfeeding, and hospital-run classes usually also

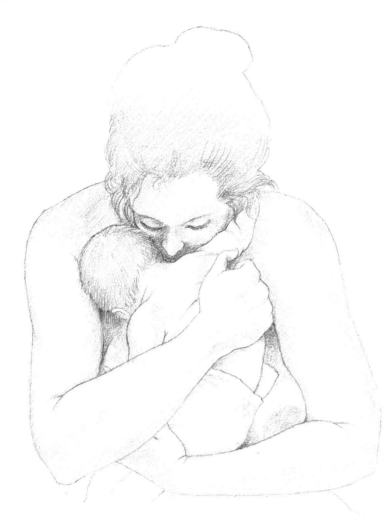

include a session, although sometimes the time is divided between breast and bottle-feeding. Although common practice, teaching all mothers-to-be to make up formula feeds contravenes the World Health Organisation Code on the Marketing of Breast Milk Substitutes.

Colette attended National Childbirth Trust classes, which included a session with the breastfeeding counsellor: *'I don't know that I learned much about feeding techniques at that time, simply because I don't think you can really take much in until you're actually doing it yourself, but I did gain a lot of confidence from her — she made breastfeeding appear very natural and easy, whereas all I had heard before that was very negative — horror stories from friends.'*

Libby feels she was typical of many first-timers: *'I was very anxious to do "nothing but the best". As far as I was concerned, I was going to breastfeed my baby and that was all there was to it. I believed it was simply a matter of choice, either to breastfeed or bottle-feed. In hospital I had many nurses trying to get Neil latched on, but without too much success — I had to give up feeding Neil entirely after a couple of weeks. Soon after, I felt rejected by Neil.*
When I discovered I was pregnant with Julia I decided I would not even try

to breastfeed her, but as time went by, I thought to myself that I might try. I continued to tell doctors and midwives that I planned to bottle-feed, though. I wanted to be left alone in my decision and to be unpressured, so I read up on breastfeeding and relaxed about the whole issue. After a wonderful birth, Julia was put to my breast, and fed well immediately. I was overjoyed! So was Julia – she wouldn't stop.'

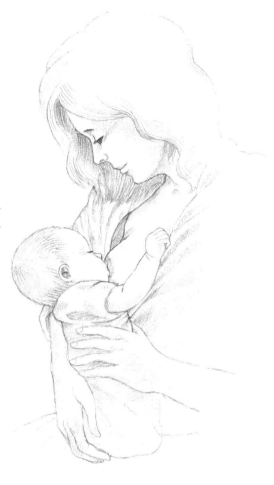

Rebecca found that classes were useful, if only to open her eyes to the reality of feeding a baby: *'I didn't listen during the Parentcraft session about "How to prepare a bottle-feed" – I was going to breastfeed, why should I need to know how to sterilise and pre-pare bottles of formula? I thought that people who bottle-fed did so because they didn't want to breastfeed, and I couldn't understand why anyone would not want to do what was best for the baby. Strangely enough, it was after a talk by an NCT breastfeeding counsellor that it first occurred to me that I might not be able to breastfeed. The counsellor mentioned that sometimes, with the best will in the world, breastfeeding does not work out for some mothers and babies. That was the first inkling I had that it just might be possible that I might not be able to breastfeed my baby.'*

Some women, Fiona included, who try to find out about breastfeed-ing before the birth feel that the information they obtain is inadequate or discouraging: *'I am currently breastfeeding my second child, now aged five months, and feel very strongly about the lack of antenatal advice about the sub-ject. Following reading and classes, I felt very well prepared for the birth itself – I felt totally unprepared for breastfeeding. Most books I looked at were illus-trated with soft focus photographs of naked mother and child engaged in breast-feeding. Although problems like cracked nipples, inadequate milk supply, were listed, the heartache and pain associated with these were never described.'*

Others, like Emma, are too preoccupied by the birth to think about what comes after it: *'Although I had attended antenatal classes, when it came to breastfeeding, I couldn't remember a thing we'd been told. My only memory was of the person giving the breastfeeding class holding a doll in her arms. I don't know whether it was my lack of concentration or her inability to keep me interested which left me so ill-informed: probably a bit of both. I know I found it very difficult to see past the birth. I wanted desperately to see my baby and make sure she or he was OK. It felt a bit like tempting fate to spend too much time and thought on preparing for life with a normal, healthy baby until I had one. So I collected up the books and leaflets on breastfeeding and took them with me to hospital, for after the birth.'*

For Moira, information was the key to success: *'I was anxious to gain as much information as possible about establishing and continuing with breast-feeding, before the arrival of the baby, believing that this would maximise my chances of breastfeeding successfully. I attended two antenatal courses, both were valuable, as they gave me the chance to ask questions about aspects of breastfeeding that I was unsure about or did not understand. Although there was some duplication of material between the two courses, I felt it was useful to hear things said by two different people with slightly different approaches, as this helped reinforce some issues that I was unclear about. Also, attending two different classes put me in touch with two groups of expectant mothers which was to prove useful in the months to come.*

One other benefit of these classes was the literature that was available, par-ticularly the NCT leaflets on breastfeeding and the handouts prepared by the breastfeeding counsellor illustrating good positioning of the baby at the breast.'

FOR MOTHER OR BABY?

YOU MAY think about starting to breastfeed because you feel you should, not really expecting to enjoy the experience; or you may look forward to it eagerly like Zoë, for yourself as well as for the baby: *'I had been looking forward to breastfeeding and had learnt all I could from books, midwives and members of the National Childbirth Trust and the Active Birth Group. I think I had wanted to breastfeed ever since I had watched my cousin feeding her baby when I was ten!'*

Gail gave priority to her baby before her own emotions: *'To be hon-*

est, I was not really looking forward to breastfeeding my baby but as an ex-paediatric nurse I knew that it was definitely the best start I could give and also the cheapest – an important point bearing in mind I was giving up work and funds would be stretched.'

From talking to others, Angela was aware that for a number of women their strongest motivation for breastfeeding is the health of the child, rather than their own satisfaction – they may even continue to breast-feed despite not enjoying it: *'It wasn't like that for me – the fact that I knew it was best for her gave me extra back-up for something that I wanted to do for myself.'*

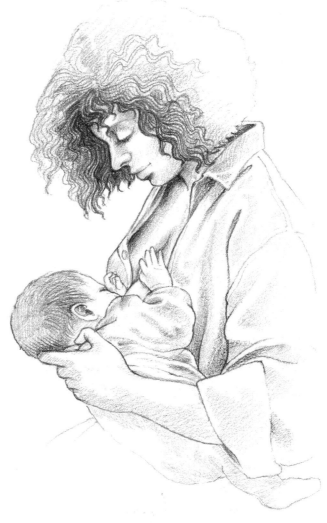

WOMEN WHO feel unsure about whether they will breast or bottle-feed may find it difficult to discuss their feelings because of the pressure they feel to breastfeed, or because no one seems ready to listen to their feelings.

Elaine found the pressure to breastfeed was over-whelming: *'I felt compelled to breastfeed. I have met several mothers who said publicly that they "couldn't" breastfeed and privately that they simply did not want to – but also that they did not wish to admit this.'*

Sometimes a policy to encourage breastfeeding can spill over into pressure, as Terri found out: *'It is what your mother did; it*

BACKGROUND NOTES

Physical changes to the breasts

The basic structure within the breasts develops at puberty. During pregnancy, the ducts (vessels down which the milk will flow) and milk-producing cells grow and multiply. The blood supply to the breasts increases, and milk begins to be made at around five months of pregnancy. You may notice very early in your pregnancy that your breasts are changing. They may become very sensitive and tender, as all the rapid development takes place.

Breasts and nipples – all shapes and sizes

Breasts and nipples alter during pregnancy. Generally, they become larger and the area around the nipple, the areola, darkens. The size of your breasts is not an important feature of breastfeeding. In other words, a woman with small breasts is just as capable of producing sufficient milk for her baby as a woman with larger breasts. The shape of your nipples is also not important. As far as the baby is concerned, it is highly unlikely that he will ever meet or feed from another pair of breasts and, to him, his mother's breasts are just perfect.

During pregnancy or soon after birth, most women's nipples tend to stand out a little from the breast. When breastfeeding, the baby takes a large 'mouthful' of your breast into his mouth and while he sucks, the nipple is drawn out more. Some nipples stand out proudly from the rest of the breast tissue, some not so much; others can be almost flat and some can be turned inwards (looking like craters). Sometimes your breasts may be viewed by a health worker while you are pregnant and you may be told that your nipples are flat or inverted and that this will make breastfeeding difficult or impossible. You may be told that you need to 'prepare' your nipples for breastfeeding. Treatments suggested may include nipple-stretching exercises, or wearing breast shells or 'Nipplettes' (both commercial devices advertised as capable of assisting the nipples to stand out). Recent research into antenatal treatments for flat or inverted nipples has established that traditional suggestions: wearing breast shells or doing nipple exercises, are not helpful. The 'Nipplette' has not been tested independently, so it is not possible to assess its usefulness. In the experience of the authors, the device has proved no more useful than any other 'remedy'.[3]

The researchers made a point of stressing that many of the mothers with inverted nipples who entered their trial had successfully established breastfeeding. The most important factor in success is to pay particular attention to making sure that the baby is effectively positioned at the breast. Once feeding well, the baby's sucking action can and does draw out flat and inverted nipples. The nipples may remain erect after feeding, or they may revert to their natural state between feeds. Some mothers find that their nipples remain permanently erect after breastfeeding.

Although many women in this trial found that their care-givers had actively discouraged them from even attempting to breastfeed because of the shape of their nipples, the modern myth that it is not possible to breastfeed with inverted nipples simply is not true.

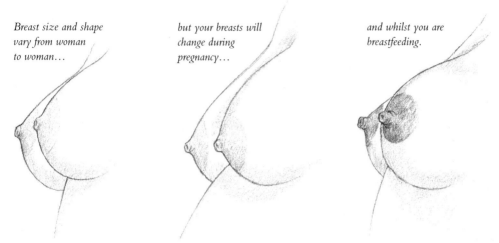

Breast size and shape vary from woman to woman...

but your breasts will change during pregnancy...

and whilst you are breastfeeding.

is what the hospital make clear to you that you ought to do. I recall sharing my feelings (about not wanting to breastfeed) with my male GP when I was 39 weeks pregnant. His advice was simple – breast milk was for babies, cow's milk for calves. I have never quite forgiven him! It's a shame that no one else could try and listen or understand how I felt at that time.'

IT IS IMPORTANT that there should be plenty of opportunity for you to discuss your feelings with a health worker or counsellor who can listen sensitively to you and who can accept what you are saying. Pregnancy and early parenthood are times of emotional upheaval which will be made more stressful if you feel unable to talk openly about your feelings without being judged.

SEX DURING PREGNANCY

PREGNANCY BRINGS changes to your breasts, and these will inevitably affect your life as a sexual couple. In the early weeks, your nipples are usually quite sensitive to touch and you may wish to avoid contact during foreplay or you may, of course, prefer more stimulation. There could be concerns about miscarriage in the early months, so you may be advised to avoid sexual intercourse altogether for some time. As the pregnancy progresses, you will need to find positions for making love that do not involve squashing the 'bump' or your breasts. Sometimes these changes bring added excitement to your relation-ship, as Karen discovered: *'When I was pregnant my husband and I enjoyed a carefree sex life, no contraception needs, no worries. I seemed to have*

FEEDING FILE

Anticipating breastfeeding together

● Attend the antenatal session on breast-feeding with your partner and discuss how you both feel about breastfeeding. Include memories, your own experiences, negative feelings and any concerns. For example: how might your partner feel about you breastfeeding in front of certain male relatives or friends? – and how do you feel?

● Expect major changes in any previous 'routines' you have developed as a couple without children

● Discuss how 'running the household' may change according to the needs of you all as a new family

● Talk to each other as much as possible about the changes you are experiencing as a pregnant woman and an expectant father. Share your imaginations (fantasies) of life after the birth – you may discover that you have similar anxieties and that you are looking forward to the same joys.

---

an increased sex drive, and he found my changing body shape exciting and stimulating. He said that in his eyes I was the most beautiful woman in the world and he found himself increasingly attracted to me far more often. This was very reassuring and made me feel very loved and wanted.'

ANTENATAL PREPARATION

SOMETIMES YOU may be told that you need to 'prepare' your nipples in some way for breastfeeding. It is not useful to 'prepare' the nipples by rubbing or scrubbing them. Nipples are sensitive because they are supposed to be sensitive. 'Toughening' them has no effect on subsequent soreness – except perhaps to worsen it. Expressing colostrum is another suggestion sometimes encountered, but is unnecessary. Unfortunately, there are still plenty of people who give this kind of advice to mothers:

'On my doctor's advice, I tried to prepare my nipples by rubbing them, first with a rough towel, later with a soft toothbrush.'

'I tried scrubbing my breasts with a washcloth after reading you should in some book, and gave up after about two minutes when I felt the pain! After that I decided I'd wait and suffer when the baby was born.'

FEEDING FILE

Preparing for breastfeeding

Your body prepares for breastfeeding whilst you are pregnant. The structure of the milk ducts and milk-producing cells develops and the blood supply to the breasts increases. Most breasts develop in size during pregnancy as a result of these changes. Some women find that, as their breasts increase in size, they are more comfortable wearing a supportive bra. It is worth remembering, though, that the actual size of your breasts does not relate in any way to their capacity for producing milk.

As pregnancy progresses, colostrum begins to be made in the breasts and this creamy-coloured substance may be noticed on the nipples. You can soak these deposits off in a warm bath if you wish. Some mothers leak colostrum in sufficient quantities to warrant wearing a breast pad. This leaking is perfectly natural, and will not 'use up' the supplies. Some women do not leak, but will still have colostrum in their breasts.

In the past, antenatal advice seemed to centre around ideas for 'toughening up' the nipples, such as scrubbing the nipples with rough towels. This is not appropriate and is very painful.

Before the birth

● Find out about breastfeeding. Clear and accurate information from a reliable, honest source is vital. Beware of 'myths' and 'old wives' tales'

● Attend antenatal classes. Most hospital classes and NCT antenatal courses include at least one session on breastfeeding

● Discuss breastfeeding with your midwife and other people who will be involved in caring for you

● All breastfeeding counsellors are happy to discuss breastfeeding at any time. NCT breastfeeding counsellors are trained to focus on the mother and her needs. They will not relate their personal experiences of breastfeeding

● Books about breastfeeding should be available at all good bookshops, and the NCT publishes leaflets on several breastfeeding topics

● Think in advance about where you will get support and encouragement once you are breastfeeding. Talking about your decision to your family and making sure they will support you can avoid conflict when the baby is born.

NATURE 'prepares' your body for birth and your breasts for breast-feeding – all you have to do is sit back and wait, and enjoy your growing, changing shape.

BACKGROUND NOTES

Why breastfeed?

In health terms breastfeeding is incomparably the best,
both for you and for your baby.

Toning your body

● Breastfeeding helps your body recover quickly from giving birth. Hormones released when your baby sucks contract your uterus a bit more each time you feed. The same hormones help to tone your muscles again

● You may find that you lose weight more quickly if you breastfeed, as breastfeeding uses up the fat stores you laid down in pregnancy.[4] In one study, women who breastfed for at least six months lost an average of 2kg more than non-breastfeeders during the first year of the baby's life. The greatest loss was in the three- to six-month period.[5] Some women only lose weight once they have finished breastfeeding

● Breastfeeding helps you to relax and feel calm – once the milk starts to flow, your hormones help you to relax and enjoy it.

Rewarding and pleasurable

● Breastfeeding brings you close to your baby. It can feel good: warm and comforting, to you as well as your baby

● Many women feel intense pleasure when their baby suckles. Others feel a great sense of pride in seeing their baby growing strong and healthy on their milk alone

● You never have to keep your baby waiting with breastfeeding. There is always milk in your breasts, and it is always instantly available.

Protecting you naturally

● Breastfeeding helps to protect you in several ways. Studies show that breastfeeding your baby for three months gives protection from breast cancer before the menopause – the risk is reduced by half.[6, 7] It also helps to protect you from ovarian cancer [8]

● Exclusive breastfeeding – that is, giving nothing but breast milk – also helps to protect you from becoming pregnant again too soon[9, 10]

● If you breastfeed, you are less at risk of osteoporosis than if you do not.[11] Although the levels of calcium in your bones do fall while you are breastfeeding, your bone mineralisation is improved and by six months after weaning, your calcium levels are higher than they would be if you had not breastfed at all

● This protection also extends to hip fractures. One study has found that women who had never breastfed had twice the risk of hip fractures than women who had breastfed. The longer you breastfeed, the greater the protection: breastfeeding for longer than nine months for each child can reduce your risk to one quarter of that of non-breastfeeders.[12]

BACKGROUND NOTES

Ideal food for your baby

● Your body has fed and protected your baby for the last nine months. Breastfeeding is designed to do the same for the next nine months

● Breast milk is the very best food your baby will ever have: it contains every nutrient your baby needs to grow and develop to her full potential.[13, 14] It even changes as your baby grows to meet her changing needs. She needs nothing else for the first four to six months.

Best for your baby's growth

● Formula milk can copy some of the basic nutrients in breast milk, but there are properties in breast milk which just cannot be copied[16, 17, 18, 19]

● Breast milk is uniquely designed to make sure that your baby's brain and central nervous system develop to their full potential

● Studies have shown that breast milk is important for the correct development of babies' eyesight, especially if they are born prematurely.[20]

Important for health

● Because your milk contains antibodies, breastfeeding is very important in helping your baby to stay healthy.[21, 22] Most importantly, breastfeeding protects your baby from dangerous stomach bugs, which cause diarrhoea. Formula-fed babies are five to ten times more likely to develop gastro-enteritis than breastfed babies[23]

● Breastfeeding also protects against breathing problems and chest infections which cause wheezing, such as bronchitis, bronchiolitis and pneumonia. Studies have found that this protection can last for several years after breastfeeding has ended[24, 25]

● Babies who are breastfed exclusively, that is with no additional formula, until at least four months of age, have been shown to suffer from half the number of ear infections of those who are never breastfed. They also have 40% fewer ear infections than those who are given supplements of formula[26, 27]

● Babies who are not exclusively breastfed for at least two months double their risk of developing insulin-dependent diabetes.[28, 29, 30]

Allergies

● Breastfeeding can help to protect your baby from allergies like eczema and asthma. It can also help to reduce the severity of these allergies if they do develop in your baby[24]

● Many experts recommend that babies from families with allergies are breastfed without any supplements for at least six months, if possible.[31]

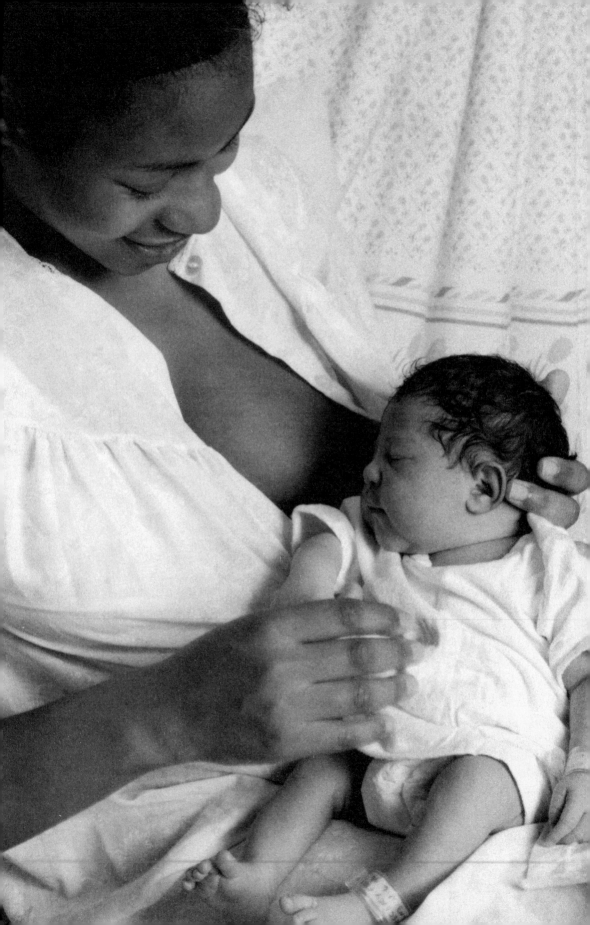

CHAPTER *<u>two</u>* The
early days

BEGINNINGS

FOR MANY mothers and babies, starting to breastfeed is straightforward, problem-free and enjoyable. You may find that your baby knows instinctively how to achieve a good meal – all you have to do is show him where it is. Ruth's baby, Laura, was wonderfully alert and was encouraged to suckle immediately: *'This was a very positive beginning. I felt so close to my baby and very much needed. She seemed to know exactly what to do. She was allowed to feed for a few minutes and I was able to feed her again once she'd had her checks and I'd been stitched up. I felt this was a treasured and rewarding initial breastfeeding experience.'*

YOUR FIRST breastfeed can produce very powerful feelings: it can be a sensual and fulfilling experience, unique to each mother, and for some almost beyond words:

'I was encouraged to put him to the breast within minutes of birth, when he sucked for just a few seconds – with the first feed I was surprised at the powerful physical and emotional feelings it produced.' Hilary's experience was simple and followed a straightforward delivery, but even if you have a more complicated delivery those first moments can be precious, as Lesley found out: *'The first time I placed our little girl on to the breast was minutes after having a caesarean section – me being flat on my back, Anne was placed on my right side, my nightdress was unbuttoned and I watched with bated breath as the midwife edged Anne towards me and teased her lips to open, and – hey presto! Anne was latched on with such speed and accuracy it was a bulls-eye first time round!*

The feelings of sheer joy and relief that the breastfeeding was going perfectly cannot be put into words – the birth had been so long and drawn out, and complicated, and interventionist, I had felt totally disempowered – but now

BACKGROUND NOTES

How breastfeeding works

There are around 15–20 milk-producing glands in the breast. Milk is made in these glands from substances absorbed from the bloodstream and stored in the milk ducts.

Making milk

Milk will be made in the breasts whether or not you breastfeed. Once the placenta is delivered, the pregnancy hormones give way to the milk-making hormone, prolactin. This hormone triggers the breasts to make milk, and also has a calming and relaxing effect on you.

The removal of milk from the breast is a critical factor in its continued production. There is a chemical in the milk which is designed to stop milk being produced if it is not used. If the milk which is made stays in the breast for too long, this chemical autocrine inhibitor – or 'suppressor' – will begin to reduce the quantity of milk produced. Babies need to feed frequently in the early weeks in order to prevent levels of this chemical suppressor building up.[32]

Once the baby starts to suckle, the hormone oxytocin is released into the bloodstream. It reaches the breasts and contracts the cells around the milk cells, forcing them to contract and pushing out the milk into the ducts. This is what some women feel as the 'let down' or milk ejection reflex: often a warm, tingling feeling. Not all women feel this reflex, though, and absence of the sensation is not an indicator that the reflex is not working.

Foremilk and hindmilk

The milk which the baby takes in a feed changes during the feed. When he first begins to suck, the baby will receive foremilk. This milk is watery to look at and is low in fat and calories, but high in the milk sugar, lac-tose. As the feed progresses, the hindmilk is released. This milk is higher in fat and calories.

Fat is very sticky. It sticks to the walls of the milk-producing cells. As the let down squeezes the milk cells, the foremilk is released first. As the feed goes on, more of the fat is forced into the ducts. As the amount of milk in the breast goes down, so the fat content goes up. At the end of the feed, the fat content is very high and it is probably this which enables the baby to decide that he has had enough.

Baby-led feeding, that is letting the baby decide when to feed, how often and for how long, ensures that he gets enough calories at each feed. If he is taken off the breast before he is ready, he may not have received enough of this high-fat, high-calorie milk. If he is swapped to the other breast too soon, he will have to take all the low-fat foremilk in that breast before he gets to the calorie-rich hind-milk again. His stomach will probably get too full before he gets enough calories.

If the baby receives too much low fat foremilk he may get very uncomfortable and 'windy'. The foremilk is very sugary and too much of it results in the breast milk passing through the baby's intestines more rapidly than usual. This means that the enzymes of the gut do not completely break down the breast milk. Consequently all the valuable food substances are not available to be absorbed. His nappies may be filled frequently with green and frothy motions and he seems fretful and always hungry. It may help to let the baby feed for as long as he wants from one breast, then if he wants to go back to the breast soon after he has finished, encourage him to feed from the same breast again. The high-fat hindmilk will help to slow down his gut and help him to feel full up.

here was something no one else could interfere with, and the two of us were doing it perfectly – just Anne and me, close, cuddling, and both relieved.'

YOU MAY wish to put your baby to the breast straight after birth. This will help the placenta to be expelled. The hormone which causes the muscle cells around the milk-producing cells to contract, 'letting down' your milk, also causes your uterus to contract.

'My second baby had fed immediately and I looked forward to this one doing the same; however there was a small problem. We had left the cord intact until it stopped pulsating and it was a very short cord. So there I was, doubled over, dangling a nipple into her mouth because she could not reach and the cord was pulling and tweaking at me from inside. Most uncomfortable!'

THERE IS GOOD evidence that babies who begin breastfeeding immediately after birth are twice as likely to still be breastfeeding at the end of a fortnight as those who begin later.[1]

It is important to note that 'putting the baby to the breast' does not necessarily mean that the baby suckled. Not all babies – or mothers – are ready to feed immediately. As yet, it is unclear how much of the benefit of early contact between you and your baby comes from the contact itself – touching, feeling, smelling and looking – and how much comes from suckling.

Jill's baby did not want to feed immediately: *'After the birth of my first baby I was a bit of a wreck. It was a very long labour with a lot of intervention – induction, epidural, forceps and episiotomy. I couldn't hold him very easily as I was still attached to all sorts of machines and was lying down, numb from the waist downwards. My partner held him, then the nurses helped me to sit up a bit and I managed to hold him and look at him and touch him. I offered him my breast and he licked it and nuzzled it, but didn't actually feed.'*

SOMETIMES THERE are medical reasons for a delay in putting the baby to the breast: you may need stitches or be recovering from an anaesthetic, or your baby may be unwell or premature. It is encouraging to note that many babies who do not feed in the first few hours after birth do go on to breastfeed successfully and happily.

Emma awoke from the general anaesthetic (for a caesarean section) to be told she had a healthy 9lb 10oz son: *'My less than enthusiastic response was, "Very nice – my tummy hurts". The next awakening was a little better, though I was still very drowsy. At least I could just about sit up in bed and hold John. I tried to feed him, but could not find a way to hold him near my breast but away from my still swollen stomach. That night, he slept in the nursery, and, with my grateful permission, was bottle-fed.*

Next morning brought a whole new meaning to life. The pain-killing injections were working, I had slept well, and felt half human. After I had a bed bath, I was asked if I wanted to try again to feed my baby. He managed his first really good feed at about 28 hours old.'

Frances didn't breastfeed her daughter, Melanie, until she was four days old: *'I had planned to bottle-feed but she wouldn't take the bottle, so my cousin suggested I try breastfeeding. One of the midwives came to help me. She was great. She helped me to get comfortable: I had a lot of stitches and had been very uncomfy when bottle-feeding. Melanie fed beautifully at once. She just took to it like a duck to water.'*

You may find that your baby, like Lisa's, is not at all interested in feeding in the early hours after delivery: *'I did not feed him in the delivery theatre, despite my intentions beforehand, as I was too dazed to get my act together (and no one suggested I should try!). A little later, in the recovery room, I asked the nurse if I should try feeding him. "You can if you like," was the reply, "but we usually bring them to you after six hours for a feed." I made an attempt to feed him but although Jack was very alert and wide-eyed for the first hour after birth, he showed no interest and, as the nurse did not seem bothered, I gave up trying and we concentrated on getting to know him in other ways.'*

POSITIONING MATTERS

RIGHT FROM THE start, taking time to position your baby well at your breast will help you to avoid becoming sore and to ensure that your baby is milking the breast effectively. Start by getting comfortable and finding out how to hold your baby comfortably at your breast. If you have had a caesarean birth or a lot of stitches, you may need to ask your midwife to help you experiment with different positions until you find one that is comfortable.

Emma tried everything, but success only came on the second day: '*I tried holding him with his feet tucked under my arm, lying on a pillow, but this was not a great success. The midwife suggested lying down, with John lying next to me, either on the bed or on a pillow. This did not work because he was too high on a pillow and was so long he still kicked my wound when laid on the bed. We next tried pillows on my tummy, holding John in the crook of my arm, which was fine until he wriggled off the pillows. Later that day, I was allowed out of bed and sitting in a chair to feed John was a great improvement. Someone found me a footstool, and this combined with about three pillows raised John high enough above my wound to be able to feed. Once he got the knack, we were away. He managed his first really good feed at about 28 hours old, and never looked back.*'

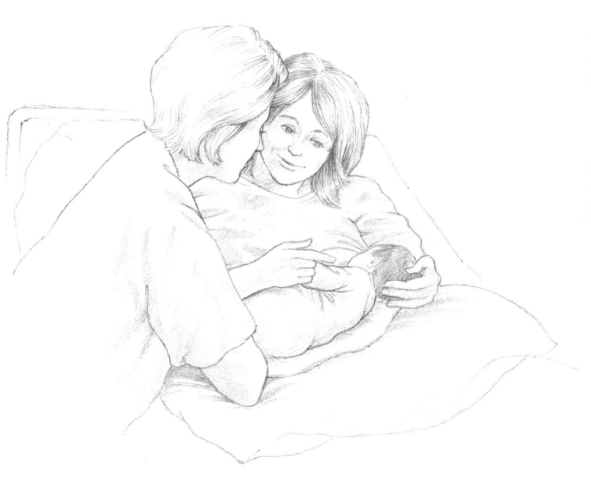

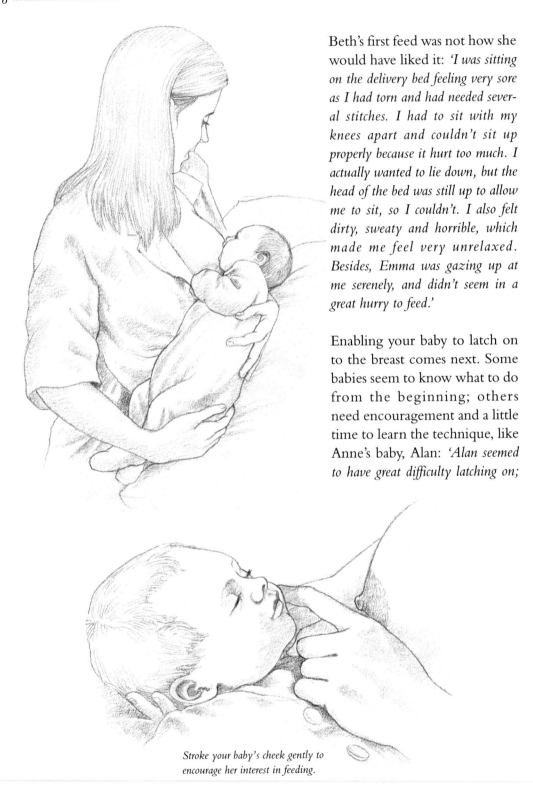

Beth's first feed was not how she would have liked it: *'I was sitting on the delivery bed feeling very sore as I had torn and had needed several stitches. I had to sit with my knees apart and couldn't sit up properly because it hurt too much. I actually wanted to lie down, but the head of the bed was still up to allow me to sit, so I couldn't. I also felt dirty, sweaty and horrible, which made me feel very unrelaxed. Besides, Emma was gazing up at me serenely, and didn't seem in a great hurry to feed.'*

Enabling your baby to latch on to the breast comes next. Some babies seem to know what to do from the beginning; others need encouragement and a little time to learn the technique, like Anne's baby, Alan: *'Alan seemed to have great difficulty latching on;*

Stroke your baby's cheek gently to encourage her interest in feeding.

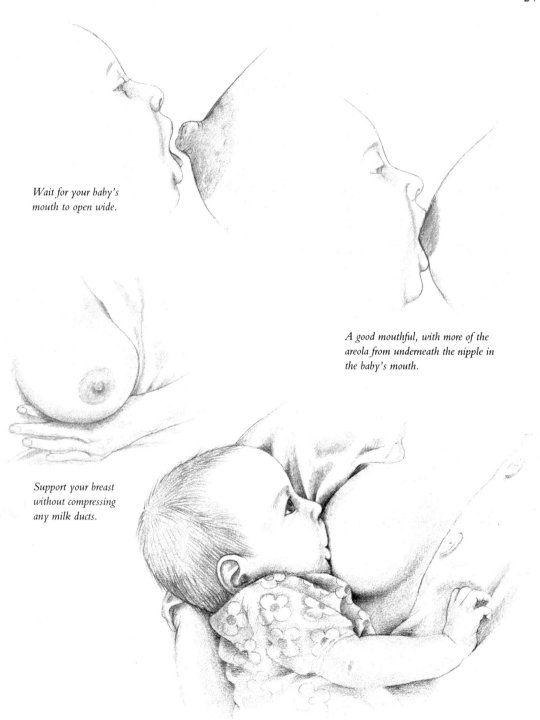

Wait for your baby's mouth to open wide.

A good mouthful, with more of the areola from underneath the nipple in the baby's mouth.

Support your breast without compressing any milk ducts.

Contented at the breast.

FEEDING FILE

LOOKING AT POSITIONING

Although breastfeeding is a natural process, it is also a skill which needs to be learned. A little attention to the detail of getting positioning right from the beginning will prevent many problems later on.

Beginning with you

Firstly, find a comfortable place to feed. Sit in a chair or lie on the bed, making sure that your back is well supported. You need to be upright, not leaning back or tipping forwards. Sitting up in bed is best avoided, as it is very difficult to get upright without slipping. It is a good idea to have a drink and perhaps a snack to hand. Many women find that they feel thirsty when the baby begins to feed.

The baby's weight should be supported with pillows, so there is no strain on your back. The baby should be facing you, with her head, neck and back in a straight line. Her head should not have to turn to reach the nipple, as this would make it very difficult for her to swallow. She needs to be positioned so that her nose is in line with your nipple, with her body tucked in close to yours. This ensures that the baby takes more of the breast tissue into her mouth from below the nipple. This is where most of the action of the baby's jaw and tongue works to strip the breast.

Latching on

Your baby may already be searching around for the nipple, but if not, her attention can be attracted by touching her lips with your nipple or stroking her cheek. It is important to wait for the baby's mouth to open wide so she can take a large mouthful of breast, with her tongue down, not on the roof of her mouth.

When, and only when, her mouth is wide open, the baby can be moved swiftly towards your breast and allowed to latch on. Be patient: she will get there. She should now have her head tilted back, with her chin stretched upwards, not tucked into her chest. Her body needs to be in line with yours, closely tucked in. She will have more of the areola from underneath the nipple in her mouth than from on top. This is because it is her tongue and lower jaw which do the work of stripping the milk from the breast. It is not necessary to force the whole areola into her mouth. As long as she took a good mouthful, that is all that matters.

It may not be necessary to hold your breast at all, but if you are more comfortable doing so, then you could hold your hand palm upwards, with your little finger against your ribcage, so that your breast rests on the flat of your hand. Alternatively, you could rest the fingers of your hand against your ribcage, with your thumb held away from the breast. This will avoid compressing any of the ducts. The 'scissor' hold, where the breast is pinched between the index and middle finger, will prevent the milk from flowing through the ducts under the fingers and could lead to a blockage.

Sucking

The baby will begin to suck strongly. At first, her sucking pattern will be regular, even, short sucks. Once the milk has let down, the

FEEDING FILE

pattern changes to a few rapid sucks, a pause, then slower, longer, drawing sucks and a swallow. As the feed progresses, she will suck, draw, swallow and pause. Pauses are a natural part of the feed, and not usually a sign that she has had enough. When she has had enough, she will release the suction and push the breast out of her mouth.

If the baby is latched on well, the sensation may well be strong, but you should not feel any pain. If it is painful, the baby's suction can be gently released by inserting a little finger into the side of her mouth. Although it is tempting to continue to feed in case it gets better, this is a mistake. It is much better to begin again and wait for the baby to offer a wide-open gape.

A good latch

If the baby seems calm and contented and you are comfortable, he is probably latched on well. Other signs to look for include: the muscles of his face working – it may even be possible to see his ears 'wiggle', although this is not always obvious; the sound of the milk being swallowed; the sensation of the milk being let down: some mothers feel a warm, tingling sensation as this happens. Only six out of ten mothers feel this, though. Most especially, your baby will be calm and content and obviously enjoying his feed.

Both breasts

It is very important to let the baby decide for himself how long he wants to stay on the first breast. Once he has had enough and has let go of the nipple, he may be moved over to the other breast. Winding is not essential, but some mothers prefer to do this. The steps to getting positioning right should be gone through once again on this side, taking time to get it right. Once the baby is latched on comfortably, allow him to feed for as long as he wants at this breast. He may only want to 'top up' at this breast. It is a good idea to start with this breast first the next time he wants to feed, to avoid getting lopsided.

Colostrum to mature milk

Once your colostrum begins to change to mature milk, the breasts may feel uncomfortably tender, hot and hard. This is because of an increased blood flow to the breasts, combined with some tissue swelling as the milk 'comes in'. If you have been feeding your baby whenever he wants, this uncomfortable fullness should only last for a short time; generally, the breasts will feel more comfortable in 24–48 hours.

After the initial fullness has passed, your breasts will probably continue to feel rather full before your baby has a feed, and softer and less full after your baby has fed. After a few weeks though, your breasts settle into providing the milk required at each feed, so you will probably not notice much difference, if any, before and after a feed. This does not mean that your milk supply has diminished in any way – just that your supply is now well established and breastfeeding is part of your life for as long as you both want it to be.

CHECKLIST

POSITIONING – HAVE I GOT IT RIGHT?

You should see:

- A relaxed and happy baby
- Chest to chest – tucked in close to you
- Chin to breast – head back and chin forward
- A wide-open mouth, with bottom lip turned out, not sucked in
- More breast in baby's mouth below nipple than above
- Face and jaw muscles working – may see 'wiggling' ears.

You should not see:

- Pinched, 'prissy' lips
- Baby's cheeks being sucked in.

You will hear:

- Sounds of milk being swallowed – a change from quick, small sucks to deeper, satisfied gulps as the milk is released from the breast.

You should not hear:

- Clicking noises
- Lip smacking.

You may feel:

- Your let down reflex working – a tingling, warm feeling
- Feelings of pleasure and enjoyment.

You should not feel:

- Pain which continues throughout the feed.

he would cry to be fed but would very quickly become frantic and even the touch of a nipple against his face did not stimulate him to suck and settle. While crying his mouth would be open wide but it would not close over the nipple; if I tried to feed him before he was actually screaming, however, he would not open his mouth wide enough to latch on properly.'

Judy found it easier: 'Right from the start he would nipple-search with a mouth that looked like a small underpass, and I'm sure that this helped enormously. There was no "snatching" to get the nipple in while his mouth was open. He would just wait for it and then clamp down.'

LET DOWN

IF YOUR baby is correctly positioned at the breast, he will first drink the sweet foremilk. As the hormone oxytocin flows in the bloodstream it causes the milk-producing cells to contract and squeeze out the hindmilk into the ducts where it is available for the baby. This squeezing of the milk down into the ducts is referred to as the let down or draught reflex. Some women experience the let down as a pleasurable sensation. Others report it as a tingling feeling and a few may feel this as pain, particularly in the early days. About 60% of women do not feel anything at all in their breasts when their hindmilk is released, but the baby thrives and receives plenty of breast milk. If you do feel a sensation, you may find it quite reassuring – if you can feel it flowing, there must be milk in your breasts. These are a few of the feelings some mothers have experienced:

'As for the let down reflex – it can be quite sharp but I didn't feel it was painful. Pleasurable? Sometimes, yes – especially if I was feeding in a relaxed way and in harmony with the baby – it adds to the feeling of nurturing, of giving life and nourishment.'

'I think the pain was caused by the let down reflex working and it did actually go on for six weeks.'

'I had expected to feel the let down reflex and experience some kind of sensation when the baby fed, but no, I felt nothing.'

'The feeling when my milk "lets down" is unlike anything I've ever experienced before. My nipples and breasts tingle and feel warm, and I get tremendous feelings of relaxation and love for my baby.'

> **BACKGROUND NOTES**
>
> ### After-pains
>
> Your uterus continues to contract at intervals after the labour is over. This lasts for a few days. Breastfeeding is a time when you might notice these 'after-pains', as the hormone which releases your milk, oxytocin, is working to contract your uterus at the same time. This is your body's way of ensuring that you get back into shape quickly.
>
> If this is your first baby, you are not likely to notice these contractions. With second or subsequent babies, they will probably be more noticeable, and you may feel a sensation rather like a period pain. Once your uterus has regained its pre-pregnancy size, the contractions will cease and the pains subside. It may help you to remember that you will be back in shape far more quickly than a mother who does not breastfeed.

UNRESTRICTED FEEDS

UNTIL FAIRLY recently it was common practice to advise mothers to feed at fixed intervals, usually four hourly, and for specific lengths of time, commonly ten minutes per side. This regime was thought to protect the baby from digestive problems due to overfeeding, and to prevent sore nipples. However, it has been shown that although some babies may be content to feed as infrequently as four hourly, this is probably only a small percentage of babies; most will ask to be fed more frequently than this, many very much more frequently. The interval between feeds is likely to vary from baby to baby and even from hour to hour for the same baby – the only constant is that there is no constant.[33] It has also been found that babies who are allowed to regulate the frequency of their feeds themselves gain weight more quickly, and are much more likely to breastfeed for a longer time than those whose feeds are restricted or timed in some way.[33]

Likewise, research has shown that limiting sucking time does not prevent sore nipples. Sore nipples are normally caused by poor positioning of the baby at the breast, rather than the sucking itself. Limiting the baby's time at the breast is actually detrimental.[34] This is because the baby needs sufficient time at the breast to obtain a balanced meal of both foremilk and hindmilk. The feed starts with lower calorie foremilk which is followed, as the volume decreases, by higher calorie hindmilk.

Fortunately, in many cases, health professionals have changed their practice in line with this research and no longer suggest restricting the frequency or duration of feeds. It is now becoming more rare to find a midwife advising a mother to limit her baby's feed in order to protect her nipples, but some mothers may still encounter this advice:

'I was encouraged to feed on demand which meant every two hours and sometimes hourly. I found this extremely tiring particularly as this was my first baby and I had a very difficult and long birth.'

'I was warned by an experienced midwife not to let him suck for longer than a few minutes on each side as this could lead to sore nipples, so I religiously prised him off after the allotted time.'

SOMETIMES, EVEN though the baby's sucking time at the breast is unrestricted, rules about the interval between feeds may be encountered in some hospitals. You may be asked to wake your baby after a certain time if she has not roused spontaneously for a feed. For a healthy full-term baby, there is rarely any need to wake her. Most mothers find that, even if they try to 'obey' the rules, their baby is not interested in co-operating until she is hungry, as Colette discovered: *'After the first little feed immediately after birth, Graham slept for six hours. The hospital sister, who was very much of the "old school", said he must not be allowed to go any longer without a feed, and insisted on waking him up by putting water on his face. She said he would be dehydrated if he didn't get some fluids. I felt at the time that this must be wrong, as he was a perfectly healthy baby, but needless to say I gave in to her "superior knowledge" and let her wake him up. I don't remember him taking more than a few sucks. I have since learned that women having second or subsequent babies in the same hospital were not treated in this way – they and their babies were left to sleep until the latter woke up.'*

SLEEPY BABIES

RESEARCH STUDIES on normal babies' feeding habits show that feeds are usually infrequent for the first few days, so some reluctance to feed at the start may be perfectly normal. Another factor contributing to a baby's refusal to suck may be the effect of pain relief during labour. Pethidine passes quickly through the placenta to the baby, and its effects can be long lasting.

Some babies who are sleepy after birth are developing jaundice. The baby's skin looks yellow and he may be reluctant to feed for very long and fall asleep after only a few sucks. Jaundice which develops at around the second to fourth day is so common that it is known as physiological jaundice. One of the best ways to reduce this type of jaundice is frequent feeding, but since jaundice can make a baby sleepy this may prove difficult. Additional fluids, such as water, may be offered in a mistaken attempt to 'flush out' the jaundice. However, the water will have no effect on the jaundice and will only serve to fill the baby's stomach so he does not want to breastfeed.

Janice was induced when she was 38 weeks pregnant after having an antepartum haemorrhage (sudden bleeding) at 36 weeks. Her baby was fine except for being a little jaundiced and very sleepy: *'I was encouraged by the hospital to give him extra fluids, mainly water, because of the jaundice, but I declined and instead we compromised with waking him to feed as frequently as possible because he was so sleepy. He progressed well once my milk supply was established and we were settled at home.'*

SOMETIMES, IF the levels of jaundice are high, the baby will be treated with phototherapy. This involves putting the baby under bright white lights, usually with his eyes covered. This reduces the jaundice, but it can also lead to the baby becoming irritable and unsettled.

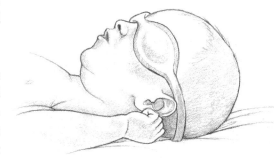

THERE IS a form of jaundice which starts towards the end of the first week of life, and may continue for several weeks. This is commonly called 'breast milk jaundice', as it seems to be found in breastfed babies with no other

BACKGROUND NOTES

JAUNDICE

During the first week of their life, many babies will become jaundiced. Most of these babies are not ill – only one baby in a thousand[35] will have something wrong with them: usually a problem with their liver or blood group incompatibility. Most jaundiced babies have 'physiological' jaundice, that is, jaundice which is caused by a natural process as the baby adapts to life outside the womb. This jaundice is harmless, rarely requires treatment and does not need to be investigated to determine the cause.

The fetus does not breathe for himself, so he needs extra red blood cells to obtain all his necessary oxygen. After birth, he breathes for himself and these extra red blood cells are no longer needed. When red blood cells are broken down by the liver, they produce bilirubin – the pigment which causes the yellow colouring of the baby's skin in jaundice.

The baby's liver is immature, and so it cannot get rid of the bilirubin quickly enough. It takes three to five days for the liver to mature, and in the meantime the bilirubin builds up and causes jaundice. Jaundice can be exacerbated by bruising at delivery; or drugs given to the mother in pregnancy or during labour (oxytocin or epidural anaesthesia).

'Early' jaundice, that is jaundice which begins in the first 24 hours of life, is an indicator that there may be a more serious cause for concern and possible medical intervention. Jaundice may also be more serious in the premature baby.

Sometimes jaundice starts a little later, towards the end of the first week of life. In the absence of any other symptoms, there is usually no cause for concern. This later jaundice is sometimes called 'breast milk' jaundice. In an otherwise healthy, thriving breastfed baby there is no reason to cause distress by taking the baby off the breast to 'diagnose' the condition, as is sometimes suggested.[35]

Is treatment necessary?

The best treatment for jaundice in a breastfed baby is to give the baby more frequent breastfeeds – around 12 feeds a day. Extra fluids, other than breast milk, are not necessary and may be harmful.[36] Jaundiced babies tend to be sleepy, so he may need to be stimulated, perhaps by changing his nappy. He may be reluctant to feed for very long for a few days, but it is important to offer the breast frequently until the jaundice passes, because your colostrum is very effective in excreting the sticky meconium in your baby's bowels. The longer the meconium stays in the bowels, the more it increases the chances of jaundice developing. Bilirubin is fat soluble, so food (especially hindmilk) helps it to be passed out more quickly; water is no good for this. If your baby is not taking very much milk, try expressing to maintain and build up your milk supply until the baby is ready to take a longer feed. The expressed milk can also be fed to the baby from a cup or spoon.

If your baby needs phototherapy, it is still important to breastfeed frequently. Do check that phototherapy is really necessary. Babies have to be placed naked under white lights (which contain the blue light which changes the bilirubin into another harmless substance). Their eyes are often covered to protect them, and babies may become unsettled and irritable under the lights, and they may develop diarrhoea. Babies under these lights will lose more water through their skin and so will need to drink more. For a breastfed baby this extra fluid can always be breast milk.

obvious symptoms except yellowness. There are several theories about what causes this, but no consensus of opinion. It used to be suggested that you should interrupt breastfeeding for 24 hours, in order to confirm the diagnosis. It is now recognised that there is no reason for doing this, as it causes distress for both mother and baby, and does not achieve very much. The levels of jaundice may fall slightly more quickly, but they will also disappear without any treatment, as Ellen's baby George's did: *'The beginning with George was uneventful – he took to breastfeeding like a duck to water and I was relaxed and confident. He was still jaundiced at four weeks and we went to hospital for blood tests. The verdict was breast milk jaundice. A pity so much blood had to be sucked out of him and so many tests, just to satisfy the medics! At least nobody suggested I should stop feeding him! By six weeks it had passed and he lost his "tan".'*

INVERTED NIPPLES

ABOUT 2% of women have inverted nipples. If your nipples look like craters and do not stand out when you are cold or during love-making, but possibly turn further inwards, then they are termed 'inverted'. Many mothers who have inverted nipples are discouraged from even trying to breastfeed. However, it must be stressed that the baby is breastfeeding, not nipple feeding: if the positioning is correct your baby should take in a good mouthful of breast. Erect nipples are useful, but not essential for breastfeeding. Given good support and help with positioning, mothers with flat or inverted nipples can breastfeed as well as anyone else, as Teresa found out: *'During my first pregnancy I felt that, for me, breastfeeding was a very important part of becoming a mum. I was strongly motivated to succeed, but warned by GPs and midwives that there may be real problems as my nipples have always been fully inverted. On a cold day I look like I have Polo mints under my sweater – complete with holes! They could not be coaxed out at all and all my massage, wearing shells and use of "Nipplettes" had absolutely no effect. I adopted a philosophical attitude – it may not be possible, but I'd do my best.*

Tim arrived two weeks early and didn't latch on easily or seem to have a very strong suck. It wasn't easy, and the hospital midwives began to doubt I had any colostrum. But before the birth slight pressure had expressed a little fluid, so I felt this was unlikely to be the case. Well-meaning midwives trying to squeeze my apparently nipple-less areolas into Tim's mouth left us both feeling tired, frustrated and did nothing for my dignity, confidence or privacy. I tried using nipple shields, which helped, and was reassured by the sight of milk in the shield at the end of a feed.

I was relieved to get home and establish regular contact with my local NCT breastfeeding counsellor. Despite pressure from midwives and health visitors to give Tim supplementary bottle-feeds, I kept these to an absolute minimum and prioritised much of my time to as much cuddling and suckling as possible.

There were times when I was very sore, tired and frustrated and I needed the support and encouragement of my husband, counsellor and friends. Our efforts were rewarded eventually as my nipples began to feel more comfortable and I realised that Tim didn't need large nipples to "suck" – he could milk the breast quite well without them.

My nipples gradually did appear during feeds – seeing light of day for the first time in my forty-one years! I was very sore and rather frightened when this process began in earnest as it was often very uncomfortable, sometimes painful, and looked alarming in its unfamiliarity. My nipples changed radically, with little skin tags hardening and eventually being shed before a more pliable, natural-looking nipple emerged for feeds. They were never erect or ready for Tim, who had to draw them out at the start of each feed.

If anyone with inverted nipples is considering NOT trying to breastfeed her baby, I would strongly advise her to think again. Like me, she may find it difficult, but the pain and heartache will soon give way to real comfort and pleasure. It's an experience I wouldn't have missed for the world.'

FULLNESS WHEN THE MILK 'COMES IN'

IF YOU FEED your baby frequently from birth, you may avoid becoming overfull as the milk comes in. If your breasts do become very full and hard (engorged) when the milk comes in, you may have particular difficulty in latching the baby on and need extra help.

When Susan's milk came in her baby had just gone to sleep after being awake and feeding for several hours, so she used the electric pump on the ward to take off just enough milk to relieve the pressure in her breasts: *'After that, if my breasts were too hard and the nipple and areola too taut for the baby to latch on, I put warm flannels on my breasts to get the milk flowing so that the nipple got softer and she could latch on.'*

Elaine had such a fierce let down that milk sprayed out everywhere at first: *'It made my breasts softer and easier to latch David on to, but my nipples were so sore it was agony. He only fed from one side and fell asleep. I changed his nappy and tried to get him to take the other side but he didn't want it and soon fell asleep again. I was left with one breast which felt like a lump of set concrete. I rang my mum and she suggested a warm bath and using flannels to soothe it. That night my milk came in and I became completely engorged. I awoke exhausted from a night of trying to latch on a screaming baby properly. I rang my mum and she came round. She suggested that I feed from the most painful side, and helped me latch David on. He fed for 30 minutes solid then fell asleep. I was still uncomfortable on the other side, with no prospect of a feed for a couple of hours — so my mum suggested that I try (unsuccessfully) to gently hand express a little, to ease the discomfort. I ended up having another warm bath coated with warm flannels.'*

Anna tried out a tip she had heard about: *'In hospital I became painfully engorged on day three and found the value in half-frozen savoy cabbage leaves — bliss when worn inside a good supportive bra and changed frequently. Not sure about the aroma, but at the time I didn't care.'*

IN MOST CASES this painful fullness passes within 24 to 48 hours, and can be eased by encouraging the milk to flow.

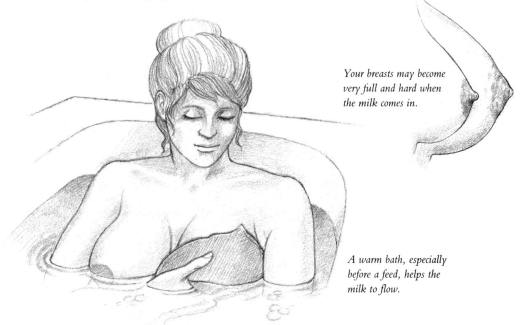

Your breasts may become very full and hard when the milk comes in.

A warm bath, especially before a feed, helps the milk to flow.

FEEDING FILE

Coping with fullness when the milk 'comes in'

Many mothers experience a change in their breasts around the third or fourth day after birth, from being soft to being firm and full. The milk is changing from colostrum to mature milk, the blood and lymph supply to your breasts has increased, and there is fluid (oedema) in your breast tissues. Your breasts may feel hot and hard, and you may experience some pain. This is often called engorgement. This is a temporary condition, which will only last for 24 to 48 hours. If you feed your baby very frequently from birth, you may avoid engorgement altogether.

How to cope

● Most importantly, feed your baby frequently, for as long as she wants

● If you are very full, you may need to soften the nipple to enable your baby to latch on. If your nipples are not standing out as much as they were, your baby may have some difficulty in taking in enough breast tissue. It would be easy to develop sore nipples if she is not taking a good mouthful

● Massage your nipples gently, and very gently push back the tissue to soften them

● Do be gentle with anything you do, as your breast tissue is easily bruised at this sensitive time

● Alternating warmth and cold can be comforting: warm flannels, a warm shower or bath, especially before a feed, helps the milk to flow; an ice-pack wrapped in a tea-towel, or even a packet of frozen peas, helps to soothe the breasts, especially after a feed

● Some mothers find that cabbage leaves which have been chilled in the fridge are soothing when slipped around the breast inside their bra. Leave them in place for half an hour or so, until they reach body temperature

● Try using a breast pump, hand or electric, just before a feed. If you become uncomfortable before your baby wants to feed again, try expressing a little milk until you feel comfortable again

● Make sure that your bra is not too tight – any constriction could lead to bruising and possibly blocked ducts or mastitis

● Ask your midwife for a suitable pain-killer such as paracetamol if you need one; this will not harm your baby.

BREASTMILK PRODUCTION FROM BIRTH				
Age of the baby	Volume per day		Volume per feed	
	Range	Average	On average	Refs.
Day 1 (0–24 hours)	7–123mls	37mls	7mls	1,3,5
Day 2 (24–48 hours)	44–335mls	84mls	14mls	3
Day 3 (48–72 hours)	98–775mls	408mls	38mls	1,2,3
Day 4 (72–96 hours)	375–876mls	625mls	58mls	1,3
Day 5 (95–120 hours)	452–876mls	700mls	70mls	1,3
3 months	609–837mls	750mls		4
6 months		800ml		

References

1. Saint, L., Smith, M. and Harmann, P. 1984: The yield and nutrient content of colostrum and milk from giving birth to one month postpartum. *British Journal of Nutrition*, vol 52: pp87-95.
2. Neville, M. et al. 1988: Studies in human lactation: milk volumes in lactating women during the onset of lactation and full lactation. *American Society for Clinical Nutrition*, vol 48: pp1375-1386.
3. Houston, M. J., Howie, P. and McNeilly, A. S. 1983: Factors affecting the duration of breastfeeding: 1. Measurement of breast milk intake in the first week of life. *Early Human Development*, vol 8: pp49-54.
4. Butte, N., Garza, C., O'Brian Smith, E. and Nichols, B. L. 1984: Human milk intake and growth in exclusively breastfed infants. *Journal of Pediatrics*, vol 104: pp187-195.
5. Roderuck, C., Williams, H. H. and Macy, J. G. 1946: *Journal of Nutrition*, vol 32: pp267-283.

© Inch & Woolridge 1995. Reproduced by kind permission.

REAL-LIFE BREASTFEEDING: THE FIRST TWO WEEKS

AT THE START of your baby's life, it can seem as if your baby is totally unpredictable. You never know when she is going to sleep and for how long, stay awake or want another feed soon. If you relax and follow your baby's lead, you will find that after a while she will begin to develop some kind of pattern. Rayanne recorded the first 14 days of her third baby Connie's life, noting when Connie fed, when she slept and when she was awake without wanting to feed. We have reproduced an example of those records below.

DAY 2

Slept from midnight to 5am, fed on and off from 5am to 8.30am, slept to 12.30pm. Fed from 12.30pm to 1.30pm, slept from 1.30pm to 3.30pm. Fed and changed at 4pm, fed again at 5pm and approx 6pm, unsettled, fed again at 7pm and finally slept until 11pm and fed on and off throughout the night whilst I slept.

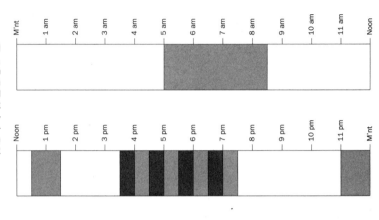

DAY 4

Fed until about 12.30am. Slept for about 10 minutes then was awake and feeding on and off most of the night in my bed. Fed at 6am and settled to sleep until 10am. Fed and was awake for a while. Bathed and fed again to settle back to sleep at about 12.30pm. Slept until 3.45pm. Fed for about half an hour. Awake, being cuddled etc. Fed again at 5.30pm for a short while, slept until 9pm. Awake, fed again at 10.15pm. Changed, fed again. Slept from 11.15pm to 2am.

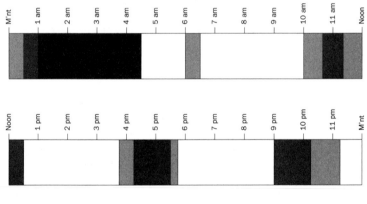

DAY 7

Fed at 2.15am. Slept until 5.45am, fed. Slept until 9am. Fed until 10am. Awake – cuddles and changing etc. Back to sleep at 11.30am. Slept until 1pm. Fed and changed. First excursion out shopping. Slept all afternoon in the buggy. Fed at 4.30pm. Changed, fed again at 5.30pm, changed, fed again at 6.30pm. Back to sleep at 7pm until 10.30pm. Fed until 11.30pm, awake.

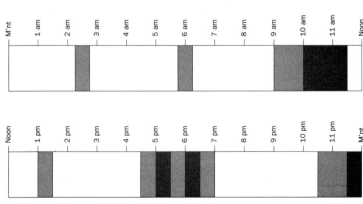

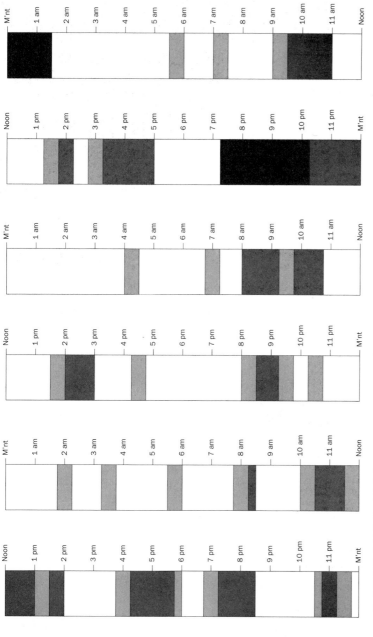

DAY 10

Slept from 1.30am until 5.30am, fed. Slept. Fed again at 7am, slept again until 9am. Fed, awake. Bathed. Settled to sleep at 11am. Slept until 1.10pm. Fed on and off for about an hour. Fed again, awake, then settled to sleep at 5pm. Slept until 7.10pm, fed, slept until 10.15pm. Fed, awake until 12.15am.

DAY 12

Woke for a feed at 4am. Fed, slept, fed again at 6.45am. Slept. Woke at 8am, dozed and cried in the car. Fed at 9.10am, changed, awake, settled to sleep at 10.45am. Woke at 1.30pm, fed, changed, awake. Dozed in car, fed at 4.10pm. Slept until 8pm. Fed, awake, fed again at 9.15pm. Slept. Changed, fed, slept at 10.45pm.

DAY 14

Slept until 1.45am. Fed, slept, fed again at 3.15am and 5.35am. Slept and fed again at 7.45am. Changed, slept from 8.30am until 10am. Fed, awake, fed again. Awake. Fed at 1pm. Awake. Slept from 2pm until 3.45pm. Fed, awake, fed again at 5.45pm. Slept from 6pm to 6.40. Fed, fell asleep at 8.30pm until 10.30pm. Fed on and off until 11.45. Settled to sleep.

KEY   SLEEP □   FEED ▨   AWAKE ▧   FEEDING & SLEEPING ■

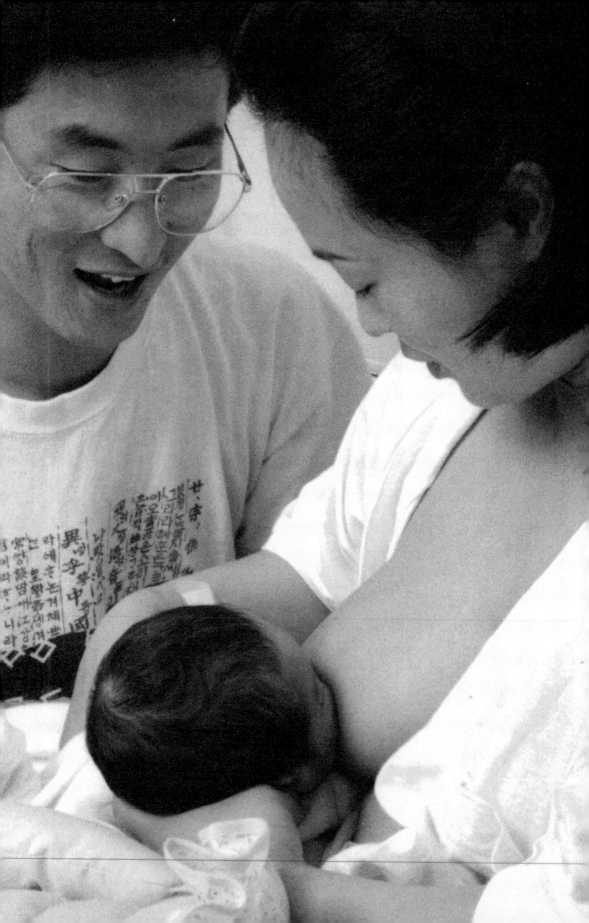

CHAPTER *three* Helping
hands

MIDWIVES IN hospitals are beginning to realise that they play a crucial role in helping a mother to get breastfeeding off to a good start. The hospital environment has perhaps not always been the best place for learning to breastfeed.[37] The UK Baby Friendly Initiative (BFI) is working to raise the awareness of good practice in hospitals. Training for all staff who meet breastfeeding mothers, establishing policies to protect and support breastfeeding, which everyone knows about – these are all important developments which are beginning to happen in maternity units all over the country. The very first maternity unit in the UK to achieve Baby Friendly status is the midwife-led unit at the Royal Bournemouth Hospital. The unit has met all of the BFI's 'ten steps to successful breastfeeding', and has raised the rate of breastfeeding on discharge from the unit to 75%.[38] This is positive proof that the attitudes and practices of staff in hospital have profound effects on the mothers who pass through their hands. If the hospital staff believe in and support breastfeeding, the mothers they meet will succeed.

A GOOD START

THERE ARE various things which help you and your baby get off to a good start with breastfeeding. One of the most important is positive support and encouragement from health professionals, friends and family. Initially, many mothers lack confidence in their ability to breastfeed successfully. They are particularly vulnerable to any unsupportive or critical comments. This is not to say that if you don't receive positive support, you are doomed to fail with breastfeeding, but it will make your task much easier if, like Gemma, you feel that those around you want you to succeed and have confidence in your ability to do so: *'There was a fantastic breastfeeding sister at the hospital at the time (who has now retired) who gave me the best possible support in the first few days. She was so calm and positive and gave me such confidence in myself and my ability to nurse my baby. She got me through a very bad case of "four day blues".'*

On the second day, Emily's baby, Huw, was fairly unsettled. Although he was her second baby and she was – at least to start with – fairly confident, she found herself wondering what she was doing wrong, rather than thinking of him as a newborn baby who might take a while to adjust to the world outside: *'Was I not giving him enough? Too much? He was definitely feeding a lot more often than the two bottle-fed babies next to us. A nurse suggested I try some water to help bring up his wind. He wasn't very interested and it didn't seem very effective. Another advised a bottle of formula: maybe the colostrum wasn't filling enough and he was hungry? I knew that the colostrum was highly nutritious and should be all that he needed, but after he'd cried on and off all the evening I was beginning to have doubts about everything. The staff and other mothers were very supportive about the crying, but they all suggested making changes to the way I was feeding Huw to stop him crying which was very undermining. I really needed someone to say "You're doing fine, don't worry, he'll settle down in due course". We left hospital on the fourth day. Huw was weighed before we went: he had regained his birth weight plus a bit, which was an enormous boost to my confidence.'*

CLEAR AND CONSISTENT INFORMATION

A SECOND KEY factor for a successful start to breastfeeding is the availability of good, clear and consistent advice and information, based on an agreed policy. Some health authorities already have such policies; others are developing them. Once a policy exists, much effort and staff training may be required to ensure that it is put into practice. It is easy to see how a mother may receive conflicting advice. It may be more difficult to avoid following it all. One suggestion is that the midwife might ask what advice you have been offered already – and by whom; or perhaps you might tell your new helper what has been said and how you felt about it. Hopefully, though, if a hospital has a clear policy for approaching breastfeeding, which they tell you about, you will not receive the confusing messages that Lydia experienced:

'The situation was not helped by the differing advice I received from each new midwife I met – often a different one at each feed. They were all extremely kind and helpful, but each had her own opinion as to the best way to approach Daniel's refusal to feed and there was no overall management plan for us to follow.'

When Joy moved from the teaching hospital to the local cottage hospital things improved a lot: *'The staff were a bit out of date on breastfeeding – they were still rather keen on four-hourly feeds, but luckily at this stage Flora did actually want to feed approximately four hourly. What was wonderful was that they all said the same thing, and they wanted me to succeed with breastfeeding.'*

Elaine received conflicting advice on the very first day: *'After David was born he was very alert and looking at me very intently. When I tried automatically to put David to my breast about 30 minutes after he had been born, one of the auxiliaries clearing up the delivery room said: "Oh, you don't want to be doing that yet – give him a chance, poor thing, he probably just wants a cuddle." I felt totally embarrassed and quickly covered myself up. I felt stupid and desperately wanted someone to help me, but I didn't dare ask. So I just sat there with tears pouring down my cheeks hugging David to me.*

About two hours later a midwife asked me whether I had fed David, she was surprised when I said that I hadn't, and told me that I could have done straight away. She helped me to latch David on. It felt strange at first, to have a slight tugging feeling at my breast, but I soon relaxed and realised I was beaming. I felt so proud of myself and my baby, it seemed the most natural thing in the world, everything and everyone else was forgotten in those first exciting minutes.'

SUPPLEMENTARY DRINKS

BREASTFED BABIES do not need any other fluids besides breast milk. Sometimes, however, additional fluids are suggested for a variety of reasons. These include thirst (and hot weather); jaundice; and hunger – either because the milk has not yet 'come in', or because breast-feeding seems to have 'failed'. None of these is a valid reason for offering formula or water – or, indeed, any other fluid. A healthy baby does not need large volumes of fluid before these become available from the breast.[33] Giving a breastfed baby anything other than

FEEDING FILE

COPING WITH CONFLICTING ADVICE

As a new mother, you may feel quite unsure about how to handle, comfort and feed your baby. Possibly you will want to ask lots of people what to do about something. It is often the case that lots of people will want to 'tell' you what to do, whether you ask or not. They want to give you advice.

Typical advice-giving statements begin with:

- 'If I were you, I'd...'
- 'When my baby was two days old, I...'
- 'If you don't do X, then Y will happen.'
- 'Stop breastfeeding now because...'
- 'It's because you are breastfeeding that...'
- 'You really ought to...'
- 'You must...'

Each one of these statements is likely to be ended with a different suggestion which can result in a new mother feeling very confused.

Tips for coping with conflicting advice

- Have an idea of how you would like to feed your baby

- Try to choose one person whom you trust, and listen to her

- Remember that you cannot be 'made' to do what you do not want for yourself or your baby

- You are the baby's mother and it is highly likely that you know your baby better than anyone else

- You do not need to try all the suggestions you are offered – try only those which seem right for you and your baby. Keep some for later and discard the rest

- Ask for an explanation of why what is being suggested might work

- If you are uneasy with advice given, ask if there is any research to support the suggestion

- If you do not feel able to listen to any more suggestions from outsiders, ask your partner, friend or relative – whoever is closest to you at the time – to shield you from it

- If you are assertive and sound confident in what you are doing, most compulsive advice-givers retreat

- It is possible that a simple 'recipe' like feeding your baby when he is hungry, comforting him when he cries and encouraging him to sleep when he is tired, could work for you

- Contact a breastfeeding counsellor. She will listen and support you in your decision making. If she does not know the answer immediately she will be able to find out and provide you with information based on current research.

breast milk in the first few days could confuse her and may in some cases lead to the end of breastfeeding. For example, in the *Infant Feeding* 1990 survey,[1] 32% of mothers whose breastfed babies also received bottles of formula milk in hospital stopped breastfeeding in the first two weeks, compared with 9% of mothers whose babies did not receive formula.

Elaine feels she was pressured into giving her baby a bottle: *'It was suggested to me by at least one midwife that David was hungry because my milk hadn't come in, and I needed my sleep, so why didn't I just let them give him a little formula to tide him over? Feeling emotionally vulnerable I fell prey to the idea that I was depriving David of something and exhausting myself in the process so I gave in during the night. I was rewarded with a very smug midwife telling me that he had guzzled down a bottle and was now sound asleep. Did I feel inadequate! Luckily that only happened once and then "the milk came in" – as if what comes before is useless!'*

Carol's experience was similar: *'The second night my nice nurse was not on, but a bossy one I was terrified of, and of course my baby woke for the night. The first part of the night we battled on – she wanted to take him away to the nursery and give him a bottle of formula. She watched me feeding, making me feel awkward and embarrassed, and said that my baby was not getting enough milk and was hungry and that I must get some rest, and stop disturbing others around me. Eventually she stormed over and wheeled my baby away for the rest of the night. I do not know to this day whether she gave him a bottle or not.'*

COLOSTRUM, THE first milk which your baby receives from the breast, may come in small quantities but it is highly nutritious and satisfying. It also contains protection from infection for the baby. A baby's stomach at birth is tiny – only about four centimetres long (about the size of a walnut) – and does not require a large quantity of milk to fill it. Nor does a newborn baby arrive starving. She has been fully nourished by the placenta, except in a very few cases.

If a baby's hunger and thirst are satisfied by other fluids, she will want to suckle less at the breast. Regular suckling at the breast, and removal of milk, is essential to help establish a good supply of breast milk. Your confidence in your ability to breastfeed is likely to be

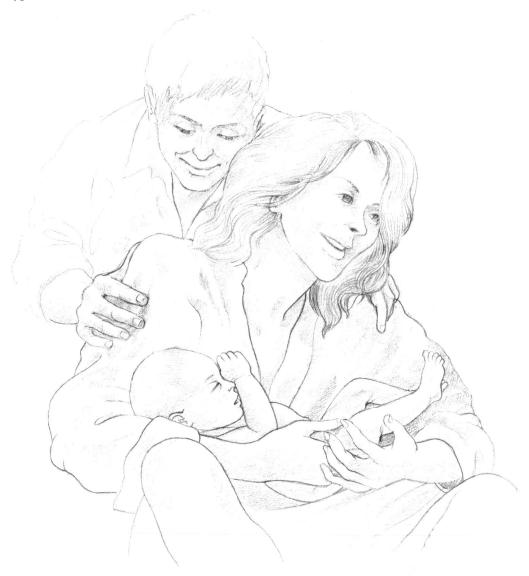

undermined if you are led to believe that your milk does not satisfy your baby's needs. In addition, the baby may find it more difficult to learn to suckle at the breast if she is also practising the very different technique of feeding from a bottle.

In the early days in hospital, if breastfeeding is becoming difficult, some women may be tempted to offer their babies the ready-made 'solution' of formula milk, as Sandra was: *'But Helen was obviously hungry and people kept on asking me if my milk had come in and telling me that sometimes it didn't come in until the fifth day after a caesarean and so I was persuaded to give her some expressed breast milk from special care — after two or three days I felt so guilty about using this that I gave her a bottle of formula. I so much wanted to breastfeed, to get something right after the perceived failure of the emergency caesarean. I knew also that giving my baby bottles might stop her from sucking properly at the breast because a bottle is so much easier to get milk from and I knew too that worry itself could stop the let down reflex. I was getting increasingly depressed. In fact, I think I spent most of the time in tears.'*

Low blood sugar

SOME HOSPITALS are concerned if a baby does not feed at regular intervals, and especially if there is a long interval between the birth and the baby's first feed. This seems to be especially worrying for the staff if the baby is heavy at birth. One concern is that the baby may become 'jittery' or hypoglycaemic. This is often the time when pressure may be brought to bear on you to give your baby a supplementary bottle of formula milk, as these three women remember with regret:

'Then the midwife said that as Alison was a very large baby (9lb 4oz), her blood sugar levels would be low and would drop further unless supplementary bottle-feeds were given. I was confused and saddened at this and merely said I didn't want to bottle-feed. The midwife did not reply and so serious did she look, I had no intention of disobeying her instructions.'

'On the second night, after 20 hours of poor feeds, Tessa's blood sugar levels were checked. I was told she needed a bottle and was undernourished. I said I wanted to breastfeed but was told it wasn't working and what was I going to do when I got home, how did I expect to care for her if I didn't even have bottles as a back-up? What little confidence I had left ebbed away. I felt an absolute failure, exceedingly tired and alone; so I reluctantly agreed for her to be taken away and fed whilst I tried to sleep.'

'My son weighed in at 5lb 14oz and I was exhausted. However, he was put to the breast straight away as I had made it clear I was going to breastfeed. I was getting lots of support (unfortunately accompanied by a lot of conflicting

---

BACKGROUND NOTES

HYPOGLYCAEMIA

Hypoglycaemia means low blood glucose concentration. For some babies this may mean they show signs of running out of 'fuel' and may become 'jittery' or start to have 'fits'. There is a small risk of damaging the brain if a baby is deprived for some time of enough 'fuel' to function. There is, however, wide disagreement amongst paediatricians about when low blood sugar is a problem for a baby.[39] This can mean that babies are tested and perhaps treated when there is no real need to do so. It seems that breastfed babies born at full term may be likely to have low blood glucose concentrations in the first few days after birth, but they can make and use other fuel in their bodies. If they are showing no symptoms, but simply have a longer interval between feeds in the first few days, they are not ill and will start to feed when they are ready.[39]

Measurement

Commonly, blood is taken from the baby's heel using a sharp needle and the drop of blood is smeared on a test reagent strip (such as BM Stix) to measure blood glucose levels. This test is designed to assess hyperglycaemia in adult diabetics and not for use in hypoglycaemia in babies, for whom it is not very accurate. The most accurate way of measuring blood glucose levels is by a laboratory blood test.

Treatment

Babies who are considered to have low blood sugar are likely to be offered additional food, often a bottle of formula or a dextrose solution. These are not necessary in most cases. Breast milk is always the best food to give, and early and frequent breastfeeding is likely to avoid problems of hypoglycaemia. If the baby is sleepy or will not feed, and there is cause for concern, expressed breast milk could be offered from a spoon or cup.

Babies who are small for dates or premature, or who are born to diabetic mothers, are more likely to need help, but even these babies may be supplemented with expressed breast milk rather than formula.

---

advice), but was by all accounts doing everything right. On the third day my son weighed only 5lb 5oz, was very miserable and started to shake uncontrollably. A blood test showed his blood sugar to be low and that supplementary bottle-feeding was essential until he regained his weight.'

SOME MOTHERS feel able to resist the pressure to give additional fluids, even though this may be strong. Tests done on the baby, commonly a heel-prick to test the baby's blood sugar levels, can become distressing for both you and your baby. It is worth asking if the tests are absolutely necessary. If the baby shows no other signs of being unwell, there is probably no need for a supplement. The best solution is to offer very frequent breastfeeds, allowing your baby to take as much as she wants from one breast before swapping to the other, ensuring that the calorie-rich hindmilk is taken. If this is not possible, supplements may be given from a cup or spoon, to avoid the baby being confused by the different sucking action of feeding from a bottle.

After 12 hours of Claudette's baby not feeding after birth, the midwife asked her if they could test Emily's blood sugar: *"'If its OK," they told me, "you will know there is no desperate panic to get her fed." The test seemed to offer the reassurance I needed, so I consented. Her blood sugar was low, but tolerable, but Emily still would not feed for more than a second. She had taken to licking colostrum off my nipples, rather than feeding properly, and this seemed to be enough to keep her going. Every two hours the midwives stuck a needle into Emily to see if her blood sugar was still dropping. I was given a chart and told that Emily must feed for at least 20 minutes every four hours if she was going to be all right. As the hours ticked by, I became more and more worried and the midwives became more and more anxious as I attempted to get her to feed. They started to mention bottles and it was hinted that Emily might be ill if she didn't feed soon. After 24 hours I was told that Emily's blood sugar was dropping and that I should give her a bottle. "Just one bottle won't do any harm," I was told. I protested that it could, but the patronising looks I got in return suggested they didn't believe me. As an aside, other girls on the ward were having similar problems and they did give their babies bottles. Of six girls, I was the only one to go home breastfeeding my baby.'*

Night feeds

BREASTFEEDS DURING the night are particularly valuable, as these feeds seem to stimulate the production of prolactin, the hormone which is involved in making breast milk, much more than feeds during the day.[40] It is commonly accepted now that babies should sleep beside their mothers, rather than in a nursery, at night. Night feeds will also help to avoid your breasts becoming overfull. You can spend time learning to latch your baby on to your breast before the milk comes in, a time when your breasts are firm and round, and perhaps less easy for the baby to manage for a time. Babies need feeding at

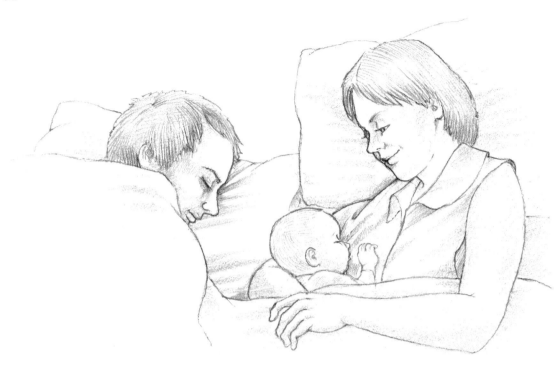

night for some weeks, and the amount of milk required will be more quickly produced if night feeding is established from the very first night. The latest *Infant Feeding* survey[1] found that by 1990, 63% of mothers had their babies with them continuously in hospital, compared with 17% in 1980. This is very much more likely to lead to mothers feeding their babies themselves at night, rather than relying on the staff to give bottles of formula. Hospital staff may offer to take the baby to the nursery on the first night, to allow you to rest after the birth. However, most mothers have already found that, by the time they give birth, a 'good night's sleep' is a fond memory. At least when you are breastfeeding, you can latch the baby on to your breast and doze while your baby feeds, and you will not be worrying whether your baby needs you. Jennifer tried this and has never looked back: *'At 2am, snuffly noises awoke me so I put on my specs and put him in bed beside me to suckle. I felt so experienced and relaxed this time, an old hand. The staff weren't bossy or pushy but just there to make sure we were OK. Richard and I fell asleep. I awoke again at 6am to find him looking up into my eyes in the half light. I immediately fell hopelessly in love. We changed sides and nodded off again.'*

HELP WITH POSITIONING

TWO OF the commonest reasons for stopping breastfeeding in the first week are the baby's refusal to suck, and painful breasts or nipples. In 1990, 36% of mothers reported having feeding problems whilst in hospital; the most common being difficulty in latching the baby on to the breast, and sore/cracked nipples. Sunita asked for as much help and advice as she needed: *'I spent most of my time in hospital with my hand on the buzzer for attention from the various midwives and helpers asking for help in fixing Jane on. I had sore nipples for two weeks – I don't know which part of me hurt more – my tail end or my nipples – it was a close thing. I was always convinced that positioning was the problem although no one seemed to really tell me what position Jane should be in, she was just "fixed on" time after time.'*

THE AVAILABILITY of skilled and experienced help for you when latching your baby on to the breast in the early days is crucial to the establishment of successful, pain-free breastfeeding. Jamie felt she

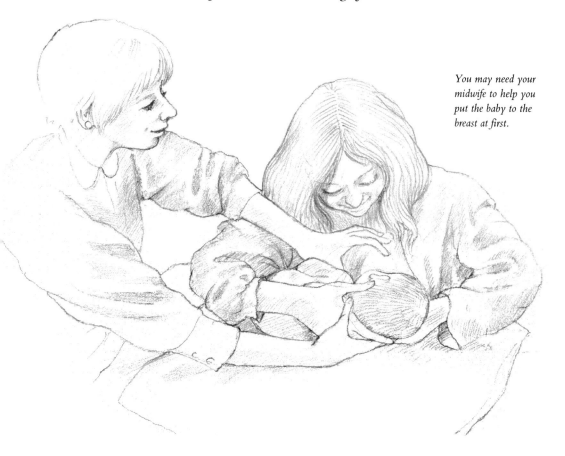

You may need your midwife to help you put the baby to the breast at first.

needed a lot of help to get Hannah latched on properly: *'She was a very sleepy baby and needed a lot of encouragement to suck. I found the nurses and midwives wonderful. They stayed with me for as long as it took to get Hannah feeding properly at nearly every feed.'*

A RELAXING ENVIRONMENT

FOR SOME mothers, the hospital environment adds to the difficulty of starting breastfeeding. With the best will in the world, hospitals are not usually places where uninterrupted peace and quiet can be made easily available. Learning a new and intimate skill such as breastfeeding is best achieved in surroundings which allow the new family to get to know each other in a quiet, relaxed environment, and where you do not have the additional 'hazard' of strangers walking in on you. Other mothers, however, are glad of the 24-hour support and are reluctant to leave hospital. Some women feel they need an 'expert' to guide them in this new role. They may not be quite ready to take on the full responsibility of motherhood, and may not feel confident in their ability to cope 'on their own'.

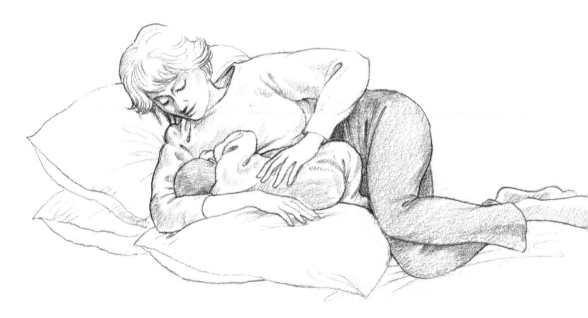

Jean found it difficult breastfeeding for the first time in a busy maternity hospital: *'The lady in the next bed was bottle-feeding her second, there were no curtains round the beds and I found it hard feeding in front of (someone else's) male visitors. Home was 100% better. Peace to feed in the comfort of your own bedroom, comfy pillows and a big bed.'*

However, Sara felt differently: *'I dreaded leaving hospital. How on earth would I manage at home, without all this care and expertise?'*

Of course, not all mothers give birth in hospital. Beginning breastfeeding at home is likely to be more peaceful and relaxed, as Ruth relates: *'When my second child was due I opted to have a home delivery. After a three-hour labour, I delivered a nine and a half pound baby girl with no intervention or drugs. The atmosphere was calm and peaceful and our sole midwife placed the baby in my arms straight away for me to discover the gender myself. After the cord had been clamped and cut and the placenta delivered, the midwife left the room to wash up. I placed the baby across my chest and latched her on myself and then shared the experience with my husband alone (our three-year-old was still sleeping).*

I then took a bath with her and she decided to feed again in the warmth of the water. I felt incredibly close to her. Afterwards we were tucked up together where she could feed on demand. It was a beautiful sunny summer's morning and the birds were singing. It couldn't have been more perfect.'

WHAT HAPPENS in the early days of breastfeeding is very important. During this first week you and your baby will have been learning together, and your breastfeeding partnership will be well under way.

BACKGROUND NOTES

A Baby-Friendly hospital?

The Baby Friendly Initiative in the UK is just a small part of the international Baby Friendly Hospital Initiative (BFHI) which was launched in 1991 by the World Health Organisation and UNICEF. There are over 3,000 hospitals worldwide which have been declared Baby Friendly – that is, they meet the criteria set out in the Ten Steps (see below) – and at the moment only two of these hospitals are in the UK.

The World Health Organisation (WHO) has estimated that worldwide around 1.5 million babies die every year because they are not breastfed.[41] The most common concerns are diarrhoeal and respiratory diseases, which are killers in the developing world, and remain the commonest reasons for babies' admission to hospital in advantaged communities.

The UK Baby Friendly Initiative has been introduced to encourage hospitals and health care facilities to adopt practices which fully promote and protect exclusive breastfeeding from birth. Baby Friendly Hospitals are recognised internationally as providers of the highest possible standards of care for breastfeeding mothers and their babies; the primary aim of the Initiative is to return breastfeeding to its rightful place as the most accepted and usual way for a mother to nourish her baby.

The BFI encourages hospitals to embrace the principles behind the Ten Steps to Successful Breastfeeding.[42] These steps aim to replace some hospital practices with an up-to-date approach based on scientific research. Several steps are easily achieved by making very slight alterations to hospital routine, and some will already be in place.

The Ten Steps to Successful Breastfeeding

● **Step One:** Having a written breastfeeding policy that is routinely communicated to all healthcare staff.

● **Step Two:** Train all healthcare staff in skills necessary to implement this policy.

● **Step Three:** Inform all pregnant women about the benefits and management of breastfeeding.

● **Step Four:** Help mothers initiate breastfeeding around an hour after birth.

● **Step Five:** Show mothers how to breastfeed and how to maintain lactation, even if they should be separated from their infants.

● **Step Six:** Give newborn infants no food or drink other than breast milk unless medically indicated.

● **Step Seven:** Practise rooming-in – allow mothers and infants to remain together – 24 hours a day.

● **Step Eight:** Encourage breastfeeding on demand.

● **Step Nine:** Give no artificial teats or pacifiers (also called dummies or soothers) to breastfeeding infants.

● **Step Ten:** Foster the establishment of breastfeeding support groups and refer mothers to them on discharge from hospital or clinic.

Further information about the UK Baby Friendly Initiative can be requested from:

The Baby Friendly Initiative
20 Guildford Street
London WC1N 1DZ
Tel: 0171 405 8400
ext. 342 Administrator
ext. 430 Andrew Radford, Director
Fax: 0171 242 0374

A MOTHERS' CHARTER

The UK Baby Friendly Initiative has published a 'Mothers' Charter' protecting breastfeeding rights. To be breastfed is the healthiest start in life an infant can have. This Charter aims to protect your right to breastfeed your baby.

A   It is your natural right to breastfeed your baby. It is your baby's natural right to be breastfed.

B   Your breast milk is tailor-made for your baby. It is specifically designed to nourish your baby, who will usually need no other form of baby food or drink in early infancy.

C   During your pregnancy you should receive up-to-date information about the health benefits of breastfeeding both to you and to your baby. Exclusive breastfeeding to four months of age has been shown to provide the maximum health benefits to you both.

D   Your midwife should discuss breastfeeding fully with you during your antenatal care. Most breastfeeding problems can be easily prevented if you receive the right advice beforehand.

E   If you plan to have your baby in hospital ask to see a copy of the hospital's policy on breastfeeding. You need to be assured that you will receive help from skilled staff when you start to breastfeed.

F   Most mothers will want to be with their babies all the time. The hospital policy should clearly state that mothers and babies can be together 24 hours a day – this is called 'rooming-in'.

G   You have a right to cuddle your baby immediately after delivery and offer the important first breastfeed. This is what your baby will instinctively want.

H   Healthcare staff should only advise that your baby be given artificial milk if it is medically necessary. In such cases the reasons should be discussed with you in full before you give your consent.

I   If you and your baby have to be separated at any time your baby should ideally receive your own expressed breast milk. Midwives will show you how to express your milk and maintain your supply.

J   Just like adults, babies like to drink different amounts at different times. Babies should be allowed to decide when to feed and for how long – this type of baby-led feeding is often called 'feeding on demand'.

K   Your right to breastfeed where and when you choose should never be questioned. No-one should make you feel uncomfortable for doing what is best for your baby.

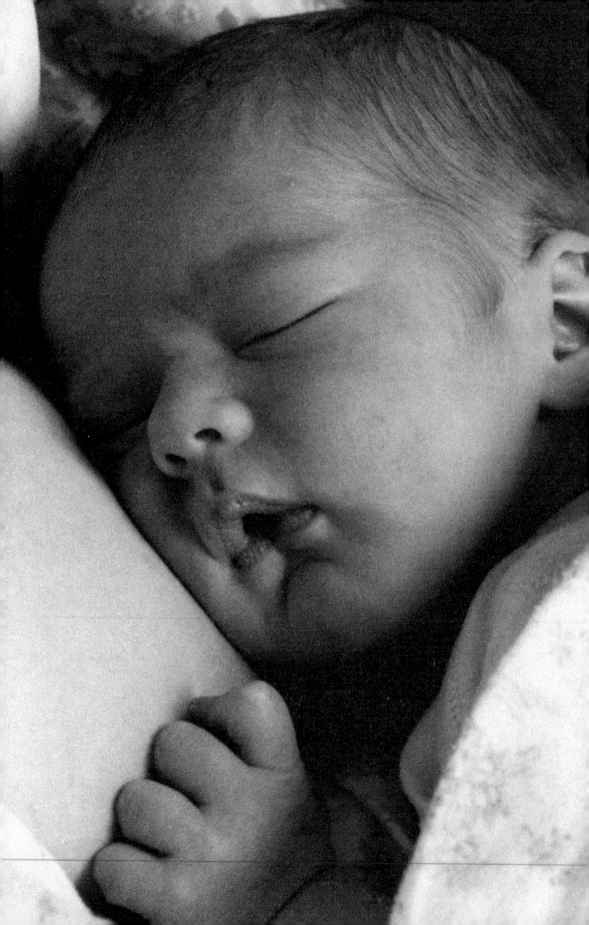

CHAPTER *four* Starting out
together

HOME SWEET HOME

GOING HOME after a hospital delivery is the beginning of a completely new phase for you and your baby. Generally, going home is a
positive step and despite some twinges of nervousness it heralds the
time when you discover how it feels to have the responsibility of caring for a new baby. If you are a first-time mother, there are usually
many different things to come to terms with.

You may be very relieved to return home, particularly if you have
not found the hospital environment conducive to relaxed breastfeeding. For most women going home is the start of getting to know their
baby more intimately.

Debbie hated being in hospital: *'The conflicting pieces of advice as the
shifts changed. The antagonism from other women (who were bottle-feeding)
who had been woken by my baby. The midwives and nurses that put their fingers in my child's mouth and gave bottles of water without my permission and
wouldn't allow me to go and sit alone in a room with my crying child at night,
telling me to get my rest. I was upset and humiliated by my lack of competence
and frustrated by the lack of control.'*

Once home, things got better and better for Claudette: *'I never timed
the feeds, their duration or frequency, and I let Eliza latch herself on, rather
than pressing her on to my breast, by just holding her in the right position.'*

Sandra found home the perfect place to enjoy getting to know her
baby: *'Breastfeeding was heavenly with my first son. I felt so very close to this
little person whose eyes would try to focus on me in that wavering, in and out
fashion. I knew I had to return to work within three months and Jacob and I
spoiled each other rotten during that time. I loved being able to catch him*

before he got fussy, I loved the noises and slurps he made, I just loved the sen-sation of nursing. I carried him constantly, breastfed him on demand and hard-ly ever put him down. You can do that with a first child. I loved lying in bed with Jacob nursing between my husband and myself. We felt so complete, just our own little world.'

AFTER GIVING birth, you may find it is quite difficult to settle down and sleep. The excitement, satisfaction and likely relief mean most women are on an 'emotional high' for some days after delivery. All this, plus the inevitability of being surrounded by other excited mothers and new babies probably means that most women return home pretty tired. The current trend is for you to be home probably about three days after an uncomplicated delivery and five or six days after a caesarean birth.

EMOTIONAL AND PRACTICAL SUPPORT

NEW MOTHERS need plenty of emotional and practical support. In the very early days at home this support may be provided by your partner, close relatives or friends.

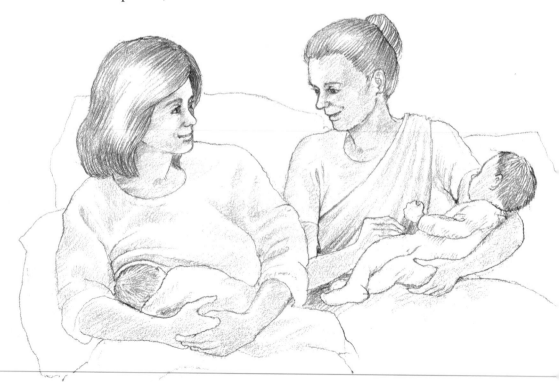

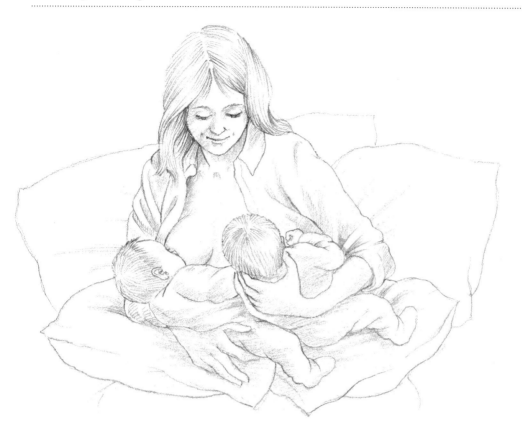

A recent survey of 115 US mothers found that 75% of these women totally breastfed when their partner approved, but less than 10% breastfed if their partner either disapproved or was indifferent.[2] Your partner, then, can be very influential. However, in such a new situation it may be difficult for some partners to discover what their most useful contribution could be. Sometimes they can get it completely wrong, as Lois found out: *'Peter gave Tessa a bottle during that first night at home. He didn't wake me when she cried, thinking that I needed the rest. By morning I had badly engorged breasts with blocked ducts. I was also terribly angry and felt redundant. I also resented Tessa being seemingly content having had a bottle. I felt even more determined not to give up breastfeeding.'*

Other women may need their husbands' strength of purpose. Ann-Marie's husband gave her just the encouragement she needed: *'I feel the biggest influence was Ivan, my husband; without his support I think I would have found it very difficult to continue breastfeeding Thomas. He supported me during my emotional outbursts of self-doubt and let it be known he believed in me. The whole picture would be totally different if at two o'clock in the morning he had been encouraging me to give a bottle.'*

For many women, the positive attitude and good memory of their partner can translate into some very valuable practical suggestions offered just at the right time. Moira's husband, Bob, reminded her of something they had learned: *'When my milk came in my breasts were very full, to the extent that Lucy could not latch on. I was quite emotional at the time and I was tired and frustrated at not being able to get my hungry baby fed. Thankfully my husband was thinking clearly at the time and, remembering some points from the NCT classes, he gently suggested I tried changing the feeding position or had a shower to help relieve some of the pressure on my breasts.'*

Some men may be able to provide more practical help than others, like Lois's partner: *'Peter then became an expert on breast massage. He did this with dedication and good humour, without embarrassment, gently and tirelessly every three hours or so for three days. Without his very special support I'm sure I would have developed mastitis and probably given up.'*

The 1990 *Infant Feeding* survey[1] found that 74% of women who were still breastfeeding at six weeks had been breastfed themselves. This suggests that a woman who has herself breastfed might be a positive, supportive role model for the new mother. Mothers and mothers-in-law are often there to help at home and give support after the baby is born, as Nicola found: *'My mother-in-law stayed with us for ten days after the birth and she had fed all five of her babies. She was very supportive, never giving advice unless I directly asked for it.'*

Other female relatives and friends who have breastfed also have a part to play, generally in offering support and encouragement. Elaine found the experiences of her sister-in-law invaluable: *'I had a visit when David was a week old, from Sally, who was breastfeeding her seven-month-old son Liam, and she suggested that I try Kamillosan ointment to soothe my nipple soreness; she lent me some and it was effective. Sally also pointed out that I could try to feed David lying down in bed, which was awkward at first with the shields but I managed. What a difference that made! I could hardly feel him suck, so the next time I attempted to take the shield off once the milk had let down, and I managed a pain-free latch. I was so relieved, at last I could really enjoy breastfeeding.'*

Gail found talking with friends and relatives who had breastfed very useful: *'I was relieved to hear that other people had also had very painful nipples and still managed to continue feeding. A friend also showed me a feeding position which helped her which looked strange but it worked. Leaning over the baby and dangling the breast into his mouth!'*

Patricia sought out other breastfeeding mothers: *'I remember needing reassurance that it was not unusual for the actual feeds to increase in length and for the intervals between feeds to decrease as the day progressed; also the pattern and timing of feeds to vary on an almost daily basis. This reassurance came from my sister-in-law and a friend who had both breastfed their children and from meeting with friends I had made during the antenatal classes, who were also breastfeeding. The mutual support of the friends with babies of the same age as Lucy definitely made the first few months of breastfeeding and motherhood easier.'*

AFTER PARTNERS, mums, mothers-in-law and female friends, health professionals are often available to offer support. Your primary care giver is your community midwife. Current practice is for her to call on you during your first ten days at home. Some years ago, the community midwife would visit every day, sometimes twice if a mother asked for that extra support, or if there was a difficulty. Recent NHS cutbacks have meant that now there is 'selective' or 'discretionary' visiting. A midwife would expect to call perhaps three or four times in those first ten days. For some women this is fine, but for others this may not be enough contact when it is most needed for establishing breastfeeding.

There is a call-out facility operating in most areas and you will be encouraged to telephone and ask for extra help if you need it. The idea seems to be that the expertise of the midwife will be directed towards those women who most need her care. This sounds very plausible, but in practice it could mean that the woman who does need the extra help may not feel able to pick up the telephone and ask. Do remember that the service is there for you to use. Your midwife will not mind you calling – she would far rather visit you than find out later that you needed her but did not ask.

Sometimes it really helps to ask for help, as Vanessa found out: *'Close to tears, I asked Nigel, my husband, to call one of the midwives who lives just around the corner. She was with me within minutes and just her presence lent some reassurance to the situation. She watched me position Rachel and confirmed that I was doing all the right things. She asked my permission to help get Rachel latched on and then gently stroked the breast to try and encourage the milk flow. Eventually having talked the whole thing through with her she suggested that perhaps Rachel wasn't hungry. What a revelation! I was greatly reassured by someone being with me and telling me that I was doing all the right things.'*

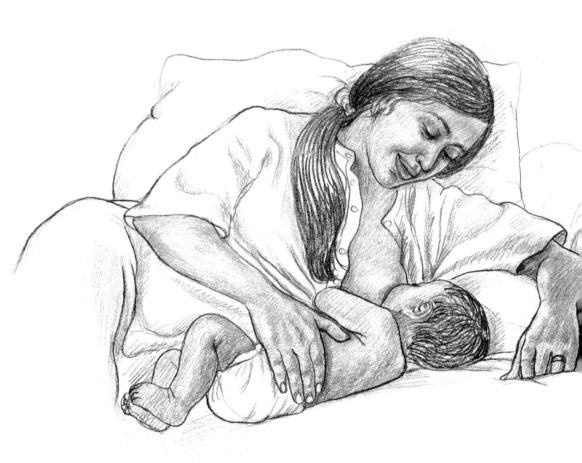

IF ALL is well, after the first ten days the community midwife will transfer the welfare of your baby to the local health visitor. Generally, the health visitor will call on you and your baby at home, explain her role and invite you to a 'well baby clinic' operating either in a local community hall or at the GP centre.

Elaine's experience of her health visitor was extremely positive: *'When my health visitor took over on the tenth day, my nipples were still sore and she was very concerned but enthusiastic about how well I had done so far. She got me to lie down on the bed and air them for thirty minutes after every feed, with plenty of towels to mop up my abundant milk supply which seemed to want to let down every five minutes! Over the next few days Joan, my health visitor, helped me to latch on properly, gradually without using the nipple shields, sitting on my bed with lots of pillows behind me supporting my back. Without Joan's constant support, encouragement and enthusiasm for my continuing to breastfeed, I think I may well have given up.'*

During this early time at home some women turn to the lay organisations, such as the National Childbirth Trust or La Leche League, for guidance:

'Once home, I became sore on my right nipple — a visit from a friend who is a breastfeeding counsellor, a cushion here, baby twizzled round "rugby" style, a closer contact, a better latch and no soreness.'

'During this time my breastfeeding counsellor was also reassuring me that I was doing all the right things and hearing from the expert really helped. Knowing she was on the end of the phone and knew of the situation was very comforting.'

NOT ALL women are as fortunate as those quoted above and the early weeks with a new baby can be a time when a mother may feel quite isolated. If your mother comes to stay to help you after your baby is born, it is possible that there could be a difference of opinion about how things 'should' be done. Feelings of isolation could arise if you wish to follow childcare practices that are different from those most popular in your mother's day. The timing of feeds and what to do when the baby cries seem to be the most contentious areas.

Mary's mother-in-law and mother had very set ideas: '*My mother-in-law told me I should put her on the bottle as my milk was too thin. My mother felt unable to advise me as she had not breastfed any of her babies, but I knew she felt I was spoiling Alex by demand feeding and trying to console her. She believed she was naughty and should be left to scream. I resented this inference that my problems were a result of my incompetence and still felt I was doing the right thing.*'

Isabel was under a lot of pressure to change the way she had started to do things: '*My husband had to go abroad for a few days so my parents came and stayed as I did not feel capable of staying on my own all day and night. My parents had very rigid ideas about bringing up a baby – you fed it and then it went back to sleep and you rocked the cradle or walked up and down with the pram until it did.*'

YOU MAY FEEL torn between doing what your mother advises as the best and doing what you feel you want to. Maybe it depends upon the

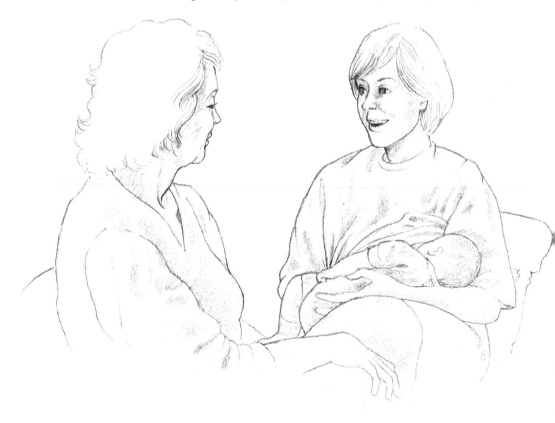

relationship already existing between you, but hopefully some sort of compromise can be reached. Talking things through and maybe explaining that you are not criticising your mother because you do not want to do things in the way she did may help.

Feelings of isolation can also arise because family members are just not available to help you; perhaps miles separate you or the burdens of earning a living give little space, time or energy for supporting a mother with a new baby.

Mary was on her own much of the time and found it hard: *'Unfortunately support from my family was non-existent partly because of distance, but thankfully my husband was understanding. But he worked shifts and had a demanding job so I was often alone with a very distressed baby and would pace the floor all night rocking her whilst he was on night duty.'*

CLEARLY GOOD support, both practical and emotional, should be provided for all mothers. A recent survey in north-east Scotland[43] has confirmed what many mothers know from experience – that tiredness and other physical or psychological problems are common after childbirth: 59% of mothers felt tired when their baby was two months old and 61% said they were unable to get as much rest as they needed. Half the mothers felt that they were not coping well when they first went home and most of these still felt this way when their babies were eight weeks old. The authors' recommendations include the reorganisation of resources to free midwives to give more time to postnatal care, and the provision of maternity aides.[43] These helpers, who would also have the role of nursery nurses, would provide continuity of care for women once they leave hospital, giving support to the mother. This is a time when you need to be selfish – look after yourself, relax and enjoy your baby: 'normal life' will still be there in the months to come. The early months of babyhood will never return.

A GOOD SUPPLY OF MILK

MAJOR CONCERNS in the early weeks and months of breastfeeding may be: 'Is my baby getting enough milk?' or 'Is she or he gaining enough weight?' These concerns may arise from your natural uncertainties as you get to know your baby or they may arise from anxieties

BACKGROUND NOTES

Weight guidelines

As a rough guide, the following weights may help you to judge your baby's weight gain or loss. It is worth trying to keep your baby in similar clothes when having him weighed, as the differences in weight are fairly small and, as you can see from these approximations, what he is wearing may make a big difference. The weights are for a six-week-old baby:

- Dry disposable nappy – approx. 1oz

- Wet disposable nappy – approx. 4oz

- Dry terry nappy – approx. 5oz

- Wet terry nappy – approx. 10oz

- Typical baby clothes: a cardigan, baby-grow, vest, wet terry nappy and plastic pants – approx. 1lb 3oz.

raised by inexperienced friends or relatives, or health professionals who might question a mother's ability to breastfeed even before she has got going.

Beth remembers her fears when her daughter was weighed before leaving hospital: *'Knowing I had to achieve a less than 10% drop in birth weight in order to be allowed home was such a pressure. Until she regained her birth weight I was terrified every time the community midwife put her on the scales, in case she said I wasn't feeding her properly.'*

At 14 days when weighed by the health visitor Anne-Marie's baby was found to have lost weight and was well below his birth weight: *'At this stage I needed a lot of reassurance and support because technically I appeared to be doing everything right. I felt very vulnerable to criticism and the "Why don't you give him a bottle?" comments and I later discovered that my husband had fielded a lot of these without letting on. I looked to my antenatal group who already had their babies and my health visitor for this support and I held a lot of store by the reassurance and support I received from my breastfeeding counsellor.'*

If early breastfeeding has not been discussed in terms of achieving a particular weight gain, visiting the baby health clinic where there does seem to be a lot of interest in the weight of the baby can come as quite a surprise as it did to Ruth: *'I was alarmed when I took Laura to the clinic for the first time at 14 days, as they said she had lost weight. I was convinced that the scales were wrong. After having a chat, the health visitor advised me to wake Laura after five hours to feed as she wasn't fitting in enough feeds in twenty-four hours. I followed her advice and the following week she had gained eight ounces – the scales were correct. The health visitor was happy. I never again had any queries about her weight gain.'*

FEEDING FILE

How to boost your milk supply

● Eat as much as you need to satisfy your hunger. Spread the food out through the 24-hour day, and maybe have a snack whenever the baby feeds

● Drink to quench your thirst, but do not force yourself to drink more than you want, as this can actually decrease your supply

● Check for effective positioning of the baby at the breast. If it hurts then seek help

● Contact the local breastfeeding counsellor and enlist her support

● Take time to concentrate on responding to your baby's need for sucking time: real 'baby-led' feeding

● Include extra 'not asked for' feeding sessions. It may be a good idea to wake your baby at night if she is sleeping for long periods of time

● Cut out any other source of sucking; this includes a dummy or bottled juice or water

● Don't organise any major social events, just for the time being

● Cut down on household chores and accept any offers of practical help

● Don't introduce a nipple shield or formula milk, as these will interfere with your supply

● Take the phone off the hook for a few hours each day and put your feet up

● If you have other children enlist the support of other mothers or willing relatives

● Maybe express milk to increase the stimulation provided for your breasts. Try dual pumping – pumping both breasts at once. Contact your local NCT branch's pump agent

● The NCT produces a range of leaflets on breastfeeding which you may find useful. Contact NCT Maternity Sales (see address on p224).

BREASTFEEDING IS, to some extent, a confidence trick: you can do it if you believe that you can. Unfortunately it seems that sometimes a poor weight gain is dealt with in ways which are likely to undermine both your confidence and your milk supply.

Anne was looking forward to the first visit to the clinic; she and her husband dressed up for the occasion: *'Don and I had speculated on the amount of weight Adrian would have gained but I remember saying: "I wish his legs weren't quite so thin." In fact when Adrian was weighed we were all shocked to find that he had lost a total of fourteen ounces on his birth weight. One of the health visitors glared at me and asked how many times a day I was*

FEEDING FILE

Cutting out complementary bottles

If you have been giving supplementary feeds of formula milk and want to cut these out, be reassured that it is possible over time.

● If you are only giving one or two small bottles over 24 hours, be bold and cut them out. Increase the number of feeds you are giving your baby and your breasts will produce more milk in response to the increased stimulation

● Ask your breastfeeding counsellor to go through positioning with you, to check that your baby is feeding efficiently

● Try the tips for increasing your milk supply

● If you are giving extra bottles at each feed, it will take a little time to cut them out altogether

● Try putting an ounce less into each bottle

● Offer the breast again after the bottle – the extra stimulation will help to boost your supply

● Cut out one bottle at a time, starting with the one you give when you seem to have most breast milk available. Take a few days over this, allowing your breasts time to build up a supply

● Once you have successfully eliminated one bottle, use the same strategy to cut out the remainder. Take your time and think positive – it can be done

● Support and encouragement from your family and friends will help, especially if your baby is temporarily more fractious while your supply is catching up with his needs.

---

feeding him and I told her five or six. They not only seemed very upset, but also gave me the feeling they thought that I had neglected Adrian on purpose. Even as I am typing this, two years on, I feel weepy about it.'

Heather had a happier, but still upsetting, experience: *'A slight hiccup worthy of note was the weekly weigh-in at the health centre. After two occasions of little weight gain I was nonchalantly told that Elizabeth had not gained the expected standard number of ounces and that I may have to consider supplementing with the bottle. However two weeks later her weight gain had doubled and far exceeded the "standard" increase.'*

THE DEFINITION of what constitutes 'appropriate' weight gain is itself open to question, since most of the growth charts currently in use are based on studies of largely bottle-fed babies conducted in the 1950s.[44, 45] Weight gain is not the only indicator of a healthy baby: if your baby is alert and responsive, and is generally happy; if she has a good skin colour, not very pale or greyish; if she is producing plenty of 'wet' nappies which do not smell; and if her stools are mustard yellow, she is almost certainly healthy.[34] Additional fluids can undermine your breastfeeding, both physically and psychologically.

It may be that in some cases there is a genuine need to boost your milk supply. The appropriate action will depend on individual circumstances.

Suzi's baby was a happy, contented, if not especially sleepy baby who seemed to gain weight very slowly: '*I decided to increase the number and lengths of feeds irrespective of whether they were demanded or not. We spent many happy hours together feeding and I look back on this time with affection. Eventually his weight began to increase steadily, the test weighing stopped and to my relief he filled out nicely.*'

Amy's little boy, Timothy, didn't gain weight very well and was fretful, and she felt that perhaps she was producing too little milk for him: '*I looked up my books and leaflets, which suggested resting more and forgetting about the housework, eating well rather than dieting as I had started to do, to get rid of the extra weight, and feeding more often. After a few weeks he was happier and began to gain more weight.*'

Anne found her health visitor was extremely encouraging and supportive: '*She told me that she had experienced very similar problems with her first baby and she was therefore able to understand only too well what I was going through. I was, and still am, eternally grateful for her support at that time. She instructed me about formula feeds, which Alan needed to get his weight up quickly. She encouraged me to continue to breastfeed as well, to attempt to increase my milk supply in the hope of being able to drop bottle feeds.*'

Maggie blames herself for her initial problems, but after some searching found the support she needed: '*Stupidly, when he started to cry and it wasn't five hours yet since his last feed, I would shove a dummy in his mouth. Within a week he lost one and a half pounds and my milk supply was nil. The health visitor told me I had lost my supply and should give him a bottle. I knew this was wrong deep down so I went to see my GP. He also told me I'd lost my milk and I would need to give him a bottle. In desperation and tears, my husband and I decided to give him a bottle – but it just didn't feel right. I wanted so badly to look like those happy breastfeeding pictures you see. My husband encouraged me to call La Leche League. I called and a fabulous woman came to my house within thirty minutes of me calling. She taught me so much. She gave me confidence I didn't have. I stopped giving him a dummy when he cried and instead put him to the breast. I fed him every hour for four days until I suddenly appeared engorged. My milk supply had increased (I've since learned that you don't lose it, it just decreases). Now when I hear people telling me to supplement with a bottle I call my La Leche League leader and get my breastfeeding mentality reality check.'*

IT MAY BE reassuring to know that some babies gain weight slowly on formula milk and have periods of unexplained crying too, as Linda found out: *'I was very sad to stop breastfeeding – I had failed and I didn't really know why. Despite being fully bottle-fed, my baby's weight gain was poor, less than half the average amount. He did vomit at each bottle feed, but this was said to be normal. Five weeks later the weight gain was still poor, the health visitor was worried and through my GP my baby was admitted to hos-*

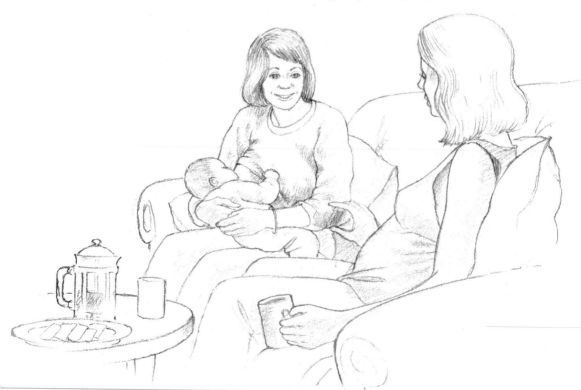

pital under observation. I really felt he was not ill, he was too alert and taking a lot of interest in his surroundings. At the end of the week the weight gain was only two ounces, they could not find anything wrong, after doing various tests, and we were sent home. At around two and a half months, weight gain became normal. I cannot understand why, when such emphasis is put on weight gain, family circumstances are not taken into account. Throughout this experience I pointed out that neither myself nor my husband have a tendency to put on weight, yet we both eat well. Both sets of grandparents have the same tendency. Surely genetics or metabolism must have been a factor to consider.'

IT IS clearly important to look at each mother and baby pair individually. Weight gain should not be the only criterion by which the 'success' of breastfeeding is judged.

GROWTH SPURTS

CHANGES IN behaviour during these early weeks of the baby's life do not always mean that you are not producing enough milk for your baby. You could simply be temporarily tense and your milk may not be so readily available to the baby when he comes to the breast.

At around five to seven weeks old, many babies suddenly increase their demand for milk, commonly referred to as a 'growth spurt'. This may take you by surprise. Your previously settled baby will suddenly ask to feed more frequently. Continuing to offer him the breast whenever he cries will quickly increase the quantity of milk available to match his new requirements. Introducing formula at this time will not allow the breast milk to increase to match the baby's new needs. Over 24–48 hours, your supply will increase to meet your baby's needs. He may continue feeding at this increased rate for a week or so, and then drop back to his previous pattern.

Elaine's patience and determination to continue breastfeeding helped her through a tense situation: *'When David was five or six weeks old he seemed to want feeding more often during the evening and at night. On one particular occasion he woke up at eleven in the evening, half an hour after I had put him down to sleep for what I thought was going to be the next three to four hours. I was exhausted and fed up and he was crying and thrashing about so that I could not get him latched on for at least twenty minutes, which*

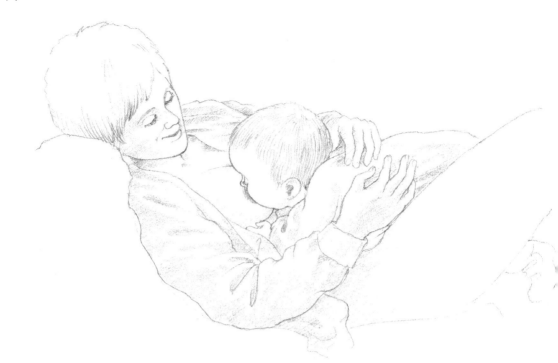

just made the situation worse. My breasts felt empty and nipples sore and I was convinced I had nothing left to give him. My husband suggested we give David a bottle of milk, which I would at that moment have loved to have done – but we didn't have any in the house. We took turns pacing the floor with a crying baby, he would doze off for ten minutes but if we tried to put him down he would wake crying again. I made myself a sandwich and a cup of tea, in an effort to "make milk" and then half an hour later I attempted to latch him on again. This time success! I practised relaxation techniques and "thought milk" which helped my prickly let down sensation and David fed for half an hour. This experience showed me how such an emotional situation filled with frustration, pain and tiredness plus a lack of information could have led to me bottle-feeding.'

TOO MUCH MILK

AT THE other end of the spectrum, some mothers and babies have difficulty with too much milk. This can be equally frustrating, particularly as many people may not recognise how awkward it can be. Joy suffered from an overabundant supply and eventually felt she had to stop breastfeeding: *'I was flooding with milk. I think the best way to*

FEEDING FILE

Tips to help with a too-plentiful milk supply

● Feed your baby whenever he wants in the early days

● It may take up to around ten weeks for the balance between the amount of milk you produce and what your baby needs to settle down

● It may be OK eventually to offer only one breast per feed

● A bra that allows one breast to be available at a time is most helpful. Breastpads can be held in place on one side whilst feeding from the other side

● Rubbing gently around the areola with ice cubes wrapped in a flannel may help the nipple to stand out

● Place a cold flannel on your breasts

● You may need to 'think milk', that is, get your milk flowing and release some of the foremilk before bringing the baby to the breast. Try to do this without using a pump, as a pump will only add to the stimulation, and may increase the amount of milk you make

● Feed your baby lying down, with her on top of you. You will probably have to support the baby's forehead. This could be called 'upside down gravity feeding'

● Be prepared to 'mop up' excess milk whilst feeding

● It may be possible to collect the milk flowing from one breast while your baby is feeding from the other breast and store it for future use, or to donate to a milk bank

● To reduce the milk flow from a breast, press gently into the breast with the heel of your hand

● If milk flows from both breasts when not required, fold your arms in front of you and gently press inwards

● Sometimes you may want to use plastic-backed breast pads if you are going out and need to protect your clothes. Do not use them all the time though, as they prevent your skin from 'breathing' and can cause soreness

● Keep a spare top with you, just in case.

describe it is – it was like someone pouring two mugs of warm water down my front every hour. I gave up after two weeks because the flooding was getting no better. I was scared to go out because I couldn't control the leakage.'

For others, like Evelyn, the flow was not quite so overwhelming: *'I found the amount of milk I had surprising. For the first four weeks or so I literally soaked with milk. I was stocking the freezer up with bottles. I thought I would never be able to go out as my clothes were drenched through every time my baby was due for a feed. Eventually, it sorted itself out to the new circumstances.'*

Practical information can often alleviate the situation, as Cath discovered: *'I turned to my local breastfeeding counsellors for assistance and they listened and supported me. It was suggested that I try to express a little foremilk immediately prior to feeding, in order to take away the first gush of milk. I also tried alternative feeding positions, including lying flat on my back with my baby on top of me, but it took about nine weeks before she was able to feed in comfort.'*

THERE IS often an overabundance of milk in the first few weeks. Generally the relationship between the amount of milk the baby requires and the amount produced by the breasts is delicately balanced and established during the first six to seven weeks, but may take around ten weeks. There are clearly exceptions to this and you will probably discover various strategies to enable you and your baby to breastfeed. It is also worth remembering that wearing drip-catching breast shells to collect the excess milk can actually make the problem worse, as they exert a constant pressure on your milk ducts, so they carry on leaking.

GROWING CONFIDENCE

IDEALLY, YOU will gently learn about yourself in your new role by interacting with your baby: cuddling, bathing and feeding her. As the days and weeks pass you will begin to feel more comfortable and confident with both the practical aspects of babycare and the emotions associated with caring for a new human being. Sophie describes how breastfeeding helped to build her confidence as a mother: *'I was still trying to gain my self-esteem as a new mother, trying to come to terms with the intensity and variety of feelings towards my baby — love and satisfaction, swiftly followed by feelings of entrapment and irritability, then feeling selfish in wanting my own life, guilt and remorse when things went wrong. To the outside world I was doing marvellously, but I felt I was failing at motherhood, doing a bad job, I was confused. Once breastfeeding was established, I found it one of the few things I did right as a mother.'*

IF YOUR natural development of confidence is interrupted by unkind, undermining comments, you may feel quite demoralised. Choosing to continue breastfeeding, even though your belief in your ability has been knocked, can be difficult. Hopefully you will be able to turn to supportive relatives and friends to help you through this time. There could well be moments, though, when despite this support, you feel it is an uphill struggle. It may help to talk to a breastfeeding counsellor too. She will have breastfed her own babies and will remember those panicky feelings when it just does not seem to be going too well. Talking with an understanding breastfeeding counsellor could be all you need to get through a bad patch.

The very special ingredient of confidence is recognised as important and enabling, something women would like to share with each other: an important ingredient for successful breastfeeding.

Gemma comments: *'If I could give a mother something it would be confidence – the confidence to relax, and confidence to know that she really is the person who knows what is best for her baby and the confidence to sift through all the "advice" she will get from all sorts of unusual sources.'*

Jill remembers: *'I learned to take everyone's comments about the quality and quantity of my milk with a large pinch of salt. But I must say it took me about eight or nine weeks to be really confident that I could feed him. If there was any advice I could give it would be BELIEVE IN YOURSELF. If you really want to do it, you can!'*

Experience brings a relaxed attitude, as Melissa discovered: *'This time as a geriatric mum with sixteen years in the NCT under my belt, I'm confident enough to do things my way. I'm much more aware of the need to eat and drink plenty and rest and let other things wait. A supportive husband who definitely thinks "breast is best" makes it so much easier – he, too, with maturity, is even more encouraging this time around. And I'm pleased to have the chance to show my elder daughter that breastfeeding is good and normal and possible.'*

YOUR CONFIDENCE grows as the baby grows. Mothers commonly experience enormous pride and happiness in the success of the relationship they have from breastfeeding their babies.

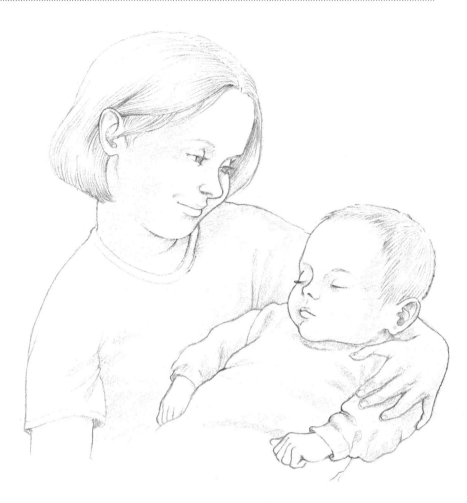

Sandra is sure that breastfeeding her baby has made all the difference to their relationship: *'I dreaded the birth of my third baby. I was so unhappy at the prospect of having another baby to care for. The unfolding of my love for her was inextricably bound to our breastfeeding together. Through breastfeeding, my love for her grew; by breastfeeding I supplied all her needs myself. I grew so proud of myself and my lovely new baby, whom I subsequently breastfed for eleven months.'*

Pam found feeding Darren an incredibly rewarding experience: *'I well remember gushes of pride and self-congratulation when I looked at him at four months and could think to myself this is all, every single cell of his body, due to my hard work. Amazing. As my confidence grew it felt great just to throw away the books and do what I felt right for myself and Darren.'*

PERHAPS THERE should be an advertising commercial on the television about this means of happiness and self-fulfilment. Is it something that breastfeeding women have been reluctant to acclaim? In a culture where breastfeeding a small baby in a restaurant might be frowned upon, perhaps it is not surprising that those who carry on and enjoy breastfeeding are reluctant to talk about the emotional satisfaction they receive from the relationship that develops between themselves and their babies.

Some people are perhaps too ready to dismiss a mother's satisfaction as somehow not important. There is plenty of news about the health benefits to you and your baby, which has been well researched. Sadly, we do not hear so much about the positive feelings women have about their capacity to breastfeed, nor how valuable a positive breastfeeding experience can be for your self-esteem.[46] There must be psychological and emotional benefits for your baby as well, in having an attentive, responsive, satisfied mother offering food and comfort from her breast.

A FLEXIBLE LIFESTYLE

SEVERAL YEARS ago, you were expected to feed small babies on a four-hourly schedule. Between the feeds, new mothers were encouraged to get on with the necessary household chores. In recent times, couples have been told to demand feed their baby. This means feeding your baby when he is hungry and not 'by the clock'. Sometimes it is called natural or baby-led feeding. In the early days, offering the baby the breast whenever he cries will encourage your breasts to develop a generous milk supply.

Thinking about this antenatally, however, can be quite difficult. The concept of the baby 'demanding' to be fed may not feel very comfortable. After all, many couples go through pregnancy assuring, or maybe convincing, themselves that the arrival of a baby will not alter their quite comfortable lifestyle. Many new parents do not want their lives altered too dramatically by the arrival of the baby. Questions like: 'How often does demand feeding mean?'; 'When will the baby go to sleep?'; 'Will there be times when life can carry on as normal?' may go through your mind. This aspect of babycare really is a step into the unknown.

FEEDING FILE

Developing new roles as parents

During the first few weeks feeding your baby may appear to monopolise your life – there may seem to be little time or energy left for anything else. You have all just become a family and it is important to give each other time to adjust to your new roles.

A role for your partner

● Ask your partner to 'field' unwanted visitors and telephone calls

● Purchase a 'baby sling' or a 'papoose-like' carrier and encourage your partner to take your baby out in it. In the colder months, a ride in the car or well-wrapped in a pram may have the same effect – giving you a break

● Ask your partner to give a bottle of expressed breast milk for a late evening feed so that you can have an early night.

Making time for each other

● Try to spend time with each other. Becoming parents involves major changes in how you see yourselves. There will be lots to talk about. Try to keep each other in touch with how you feel as individuals and as a couple

● If you would like to go out together without your baby, arrange for a well-known and trusted carer to babysit. You could leave a bottle of expressed breast milk, or breastfeed just before leaving and immediately on return

● Retain and value your sense of humour

● Exchange a dose of 'Tender Loving Care' at very regular intervals.

Each baby is a unique individual with his or her own special feeding needs, as Barbara gradually learned to accept: *'I never knew, from one day to the next, when she would be awake or asleep, or when she would want to feed. At first I found this very difficult. I was always not having a shower or not starting to write a letter because she might wake, then she would sleep on for ages and I'd done nothing. With time, I got used to doing things in short bursts, with the occasional longer stretch. Breastfeeding was a great advantage because when she woke I could feed her at once and I didn't have to make time for preparing bottles and sterilising. I spent countless hours feeding her, daydreaming or reading a book.'*

Sometimes it is hard to imagine what it will actually be like to breast-feed and, like Evelyn, you may take a little while to adjust: *'I never appreciated what a commitment breastfeeding was until I did it. If your baby has no particular routine you have to be around twenty-four hours a day to feed. I have vivid memories of trying to do Christmas shopping when my daughter was three and a half months old and phoning home every half hour to make sure she wasn't screaming for food. I did express milk for her into a bottle which she would drink if hungry, but I also found that if I was away for more than three to four hours at a time my breasts would become really full and uncomfortable.'*

Ruth had the memory of feeding her first daughter to encourage her: *'For the first three or four months of Mary's life I never knew where I was with the feeding, no two days were the same. I never felt I could leave Mary. I didn't know when she would need a feed. There were times when I felt very resentful, like a feeding machine. I felt tied and desperately tired. It was at this time that I could understand a woman wanting to abandon breastfeeding. I was determined to continue. I feel that the memory of feeding Laura successfully encouraged me to keep going.'*

Sally followed her baby's lead: *'After the first few weeks where he'd feed mostly three-hourly, his pattern changed a little and sometimes he'd go four hours, sometimes only two, but after a while I stopped looking at the clock and was much happier then. After all it didn't really matter if we were both happy.'*

IN ORDER to maintain the baby's milk supply, your breasts need to be stimulated quite frequently. Fortunately, small babies enjoy their time at the breast and allowing your baby free access to your breasts ensures that plenty of milk will be there for him. Sometimes he may take a small 'snack' from the breasts; at other times he will want to spend much longer feeding, taking both the foremilk and the fat-rich hindmilk. Rather like adults: sometimes we fancy a sandwich, other times we prefer a three-course meal. A baby's stomach is very small, so physically it just cannot hold very large quantities. During a 24-hour period your baby will take a combination of 'short' and 'long' feeds. He will regulate his own appetite, taking just what he needs when he needs it. Over the weeks some babies do seem to develop their own patterns of feeding and you will begin to recognise what these patterns are, as these mothers did:

'My first baby fed continuously throughout his twelve-hour days, but slept through the night from an early age. My second fed so quickly and infrequently (more or less four hourly!) that I thought there was something wrong. Number three was similar to number two.'

'Alex fed frequently and it always seemed easier to feed her than to devise alternative methods of distraction. At about six weeks I remember a visit from a friend with her first baby, born a few days before Alex. Her son fed once while I managed to slot in about three feeds.'

FEW BABIES adopt a definite, repeating pattern that can be relied upon. This means that each day could be different. Your baby may need more food or comfort than the day before, so if you are expecting him to be the same today as he was yesterday, you will be surprised.

There could be periods in a day when it seems as though your baby does not really know what he wants and you can try lots of different strategies to comfort him only to find that nothing works for any appreciable length of time. These are the frustrations felt during the early days as mother and baby learn to understand one another. Perhaps it is fair to comment that as the days pass into weeks most parents begin to understand and interpret their baby's cries quite accurately.

Demand feeding can work both ways. You can encourage your baby to feed when the baby has not asked to do so. For example, if you wish to leave your baby or visit somewhere where you do not expect it to be convenient for you to breastfeed, you could offer the baby a feed beforehand so that he is 'full up' whilst you are out or not available.

FEEDING AND SLEEPING

SMALL BABIES do not recognise the distinction between night and day. There is no day and night in the womb. In fact many pregnant women find that their baby is quite active when they settle down for a night's sleep. For the baby then, feeding must be an event that occurs whenever it is needed, regardless of the time of day or night.

As your milk supply is building up to meet the baby's requirements, your breasts will become extremely uncomfortable if your baby does not feed. The milk-making hormone prolactin is present in the bloodstream in greater quantities at night, so night suckling is really good for building up and keeping a good supply of milk.

Responding quickly to the cries of your baby, and keeping her close to you will mean that she can be fed with the minimum of disturbance. Gradually, she will pick up cues from you and learn that night hours are not for socialising. The time and frequency of night feeds is very individual.

Some mothers, like Lucy, find that their babies sleep through the night at a very early age: *'She slept through the night from about eleven o'clock to six in the morning from four weeks, and her night gradually got longer.'*

Having a baby who sleeps through the night can cause problems though, as Helen found: *'At around eight months bedtime became easier, but he still wanted fairly frequent breastfeeds, usually every couple of hours. Although the last feed was around eight in the evening, by eleven o'clock, I was getting uncomfortably full, so before I went to bed I would lift the baby out of the cot, feed him and put him back. It was as if he had not been disturbed.'*

Some babies take a lot longer to settle into a clear distinction of daytime and night-time behaviour, like Elaine's baby: *'David continued to feed frequently throughout the night and I think that I would have been concerned about him if I had not had Jenny as a role model. Her baby just fed all night and there was quite obviously nothing wrong with him.'*

CONSTANT NIGHT waking is tiring and it can be a source of distress. Some couples accept it easily and adjust their own sleeping patterns to allow for the tiredness they may experience, perhaps settling down for the night a little earlier, or taking a nap during the day sometimes.

It seems as though some parents believe that the reason for the waking is intrinsically linked with the way they feed their baby. It is true that breast milk is more easily digested than formula milk and therefore some breastfed babies will ask to feed frequently.

For Jane, this fact came to her attention too late: *'No one told me that breast milk digests more quickly than bottle milk so a baby is less likely to sleep through the night. I feel totally pissed off with getting up at night at least once and never knowing how long it will be till I wake up to a baby's crying. I feel chained to the baby and boobs – we can never be more than three hours apart.'*

THOSE BABIES fed on formula milk will perhaps 'go longer between feeds' but it cannot be assumed that a baby will automatically change his feeding needs if he were to stop breastfeeding. Some women introduce formula believing and hoping that if they do so their baby will 'go longer between feeds' or 'sleep through'. Sometimes the first few formula feeds may bring that effect as the baby's stomach is not accustomed to the different composition of the milk. Often, the quantity of formula milk will need to be increased to maintain the effect. In some cases, adding formula milk has no effect on the baby's sleeping habits and for some it can lead to an upset stomach and so greater night time disturbance. There is no guarantee that formula will change your baby's habits, but Colette reckons she has been tempted to try it: *'From my completely random and unscientific study of friends and acquaintances with young babies, I am convinced that bottle-fed babies do sleep better – there are of course bottle-fed babies who are bad sleepers, but nearly all of the good sleepers are bottle-fed. I know that this is because formula milk is said to be harder to digest than breast milk, with the result that the bottle-fed baby lasts longer between feeds and I also know that breastfeeding counsellors would argue that breast milk is so much better for a baby than formula milk that all the broken nights are worthwhile. After eight months of broken nights, I am not convinced!'*

LEARNING TO LIVE WITH FLEXIBILITY

ONE OF THE challenges of being a parent is to adjust to the changing ways of children as they grow and develop, regardless of how they are fed. People may live fairly regulated lives before becoming parents and adjusting to the flexible nature of a baby may not be easy.

Perhaps the most difficult change to accept is the feeling of not being in control of how a day will turn out. Many adults strive to 'be in control' of their lives, perhaps thinking that being in control is the route to coping successfully with life. Babies, on the other hand, are not in control of anything. They express their needs as and when they occur, quite vociferously at times. While looking after a new baby, you may begin to wonder when you will manage to be 'in control' of the baby and your lives again.

Parents of older children acknowledge their children as totally separate individuals very easily. They know from experience that they do not 'control' their children. Perhaps it would be easier all round if there was an acknowledgement as soon as a new baby is born that parents are not intended to 'control' their babies. This acceptance would save the heartache and battles associated with parents striving to 'get the baby into a routine' long before it is possible or appropriate to do so.

Sunita would be the first to say that having children has taught her a lot about basic human psychology: *'After all, who says babies and toddlers don't need to feed at night – do we have telepathic insight into what our children need? Are we dictating our children's behaviour or do we allow them to have minds of their own? Surely they are the best judge of what they need and don't need, and a fulfilled need is one that goes away. Children are little for such a short time of our lives I believe we owe it to them to satisfy those needs.'*

Getting to know your baby and trying to learn how to respond to his needs, free from the expectations of routine or the pressure of trying to be in control, can be a joyful and fulfilling experience, as Carly agrees: *'I'm a bit of a breastfeeding junkie. At the end of a long day (and some days are very long!) she lies soothed in my arms as she strokes my skin, her eyes close and she becomes totally satisfied and peaceful. I stroke her brow and her soft chubby cheeks and think I know why this symbiotic relationship is the ultimate nurturing experience.'*

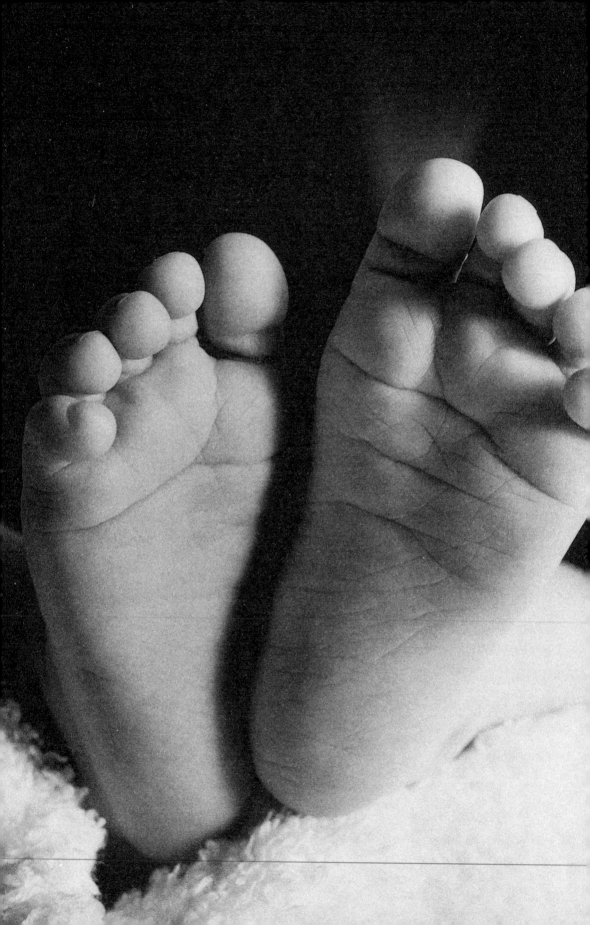

CHAPTER *five* Stepping out with confidence

GETTING AROUND WITH YOUR BABY

AFTER THE initial weeks of learning to breastfeed, most mothers wish to resume a semblance of 'normal' life. This means that you will need to be capable and comfortable feeding your baby when strangers are around, and when you are out of the house. For some women, the first hurdle to this will be feeding in front of visitors in your own home.

Judy's first experience of how embarrassed other people may feel led to a lot of confusion: *'The meal was on the hob simmering and requiring the occasional stir. My baby son decided that he wished to be fed so I proceeded to offer him the breast. At which point the guests all decided to try and find something to read on the wall in order to divert their gaze, and were relieved to realise they could go and look around the garden. My husband followed with much bewilderment wondering what had caused the stampede. I was left with no one to talk to, and a meal which might burn. At this point I should explain that my baby is tongue-tied and although able to breastfeed, he was not able to create any suction. The slightest movement by me would take him off the breast and disturb his peaceful feed. Finally my first son returned to find out if I was all right. I have to admit to feeling more than irritated by the situation, and asked him to get my husband to watch the meal. There was then a farcical situation with the relatives outside, me inside breastfeeding, my husband cooking. When the feed was finished, I put the little one to bed. As soon as my relatives realised I was fully covered they made a bee-line back to the house and the sofas.'*

FOR SOME women there seem to be two main areas of concern. Firstly, 'Will I be able to do it?' which could be translated into 'Can I bare my breasts in public?' and secondly, 'What will other people's reactions be?' which could be translated into 'Will I suffer any embarrassing moments?'

Breastfeeding in public was initially a great concern to Lesley: *'I found it extremely helpful to be with women who were also breastfeeding from my NCT group, and so my first experiences were very positive and relaxed. When Laura and I ventured out into the big wide world, it wasn't a problem, discretion always being my motto, but no way was I feeding Laura in shop toilets. I quickly learnt the "baby-friendly" shops with appropriate facilities and geared shopping expeditions around them.'*

When it came to feeding her baby in front of other people, Angela did sometimes feel a bit self-conscious: *'But I also hoped that I was perhaps in a small way helping to break down barriers for others – the more women that are visibly feeding in public the more acceptable it becomes, so long as they are sensitive to other people's feelings. Maybe I was also proud of my breasts at last.'*

Sometimes more senior members of the family or older friends can help you gain in confidence about breastfeeding away from your own home. Tracy was pleased to find this was the case: *'I can recall visiting my grandparents-in-law with my first child, about six weeks old, who were horrified when my husband suggested I should go upstairs to feed her. I was really glad that they were so supportive. (They are both in their eighties.)'*

Sadly not all grandparents are as supportive, as Zoë discovered: *'At Katy's feeds I was supposed to go upstairs to spare Grandpa any embarrassment but as she fed frequently in the evenings, it was lonely upstairs – I felt stigmatised. However we did reach a compromise – I was allowed in the lounge with my chair turned to the wall! I am surprised by how I still feel angry about this attitude.'*

IT IS QUITE likely that you will not experience any anxiety at all about feeding outside your own home. Once you have established breastfeeding you may find being unable to respond to your baby's cries for food quite distressing. You may also experience the sensations associated with letting your milk down. This is a reflex action which is usually an efficient means of the milk being readily available for your baby. The baby crying triggers the reflex, which responds by letting the milk down. Knowing you can pacify your baby simply and quickly means that you will probably find you want to breastfeed when you are out and about even if you have had previous worries. As any new parents know, a crying baby is likely to be more noticeable than one quietly enjoying his feed.

Kath was always a very private feeder: *'My outside experiences are few, once in the foyer of a motorway service station (I couldn't afford to eat in the restaurant – we hadn't been asked to leave), once in a Dorset field after a so-called fun run. I didn't feed away from home very often unless I was in someone's house. No one ever suggested that I should stop or do it elsewhere, even when I was in a non-breastfeeding house. I would have been mortified if they*

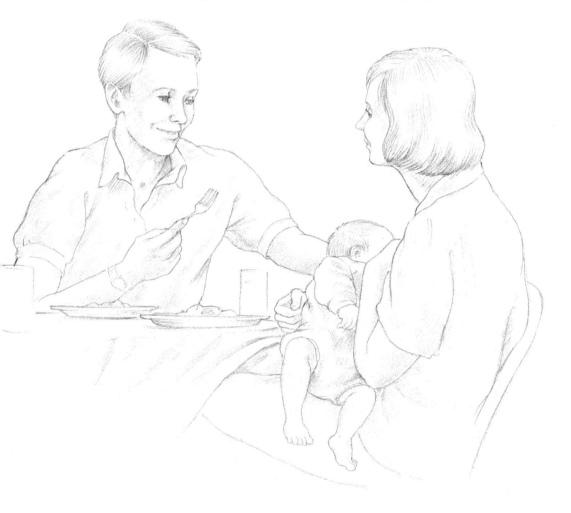

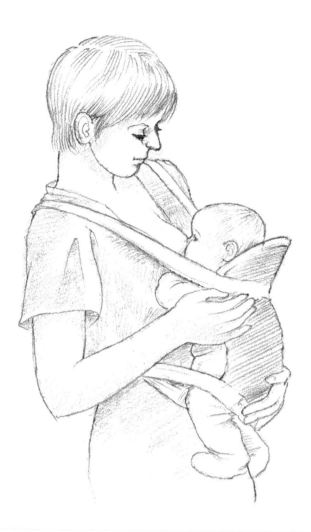

had! It used to cross my mind, what if someone asks me to move? What will I do? Nothing, in the event, because no one did glare or tut or complain. Which makes me realise that lots of babies are being breastfed out there but because it is easy and calm and quiet no one notices.'

For mothers of twins discreet breastfeeding may not be an option, though, as Ella describes: *'Next came going out (one can't remain a hermit because you've got twins). Friends would invite us over for meals and we'd request a sofa and two pillows at the ready. It was usually – Hi, how are you? and where's the sofa, you don't mind do you? Up with the jumper and out with the boobs. There was no way you could be modest or discreet until the babies were latched on and then possibly you could do a slight pull down of the jumper. Going out shopping was fitted in between feeds, there really aren't too many places you can breastfeed twins in public, unless I did them separately which would then throw them out of routine for the rest of the day. We went away on holiday whilst breastfeeding and flights don't always fit into babies' schedules, so we had introduced the odd bottle in during the day. We juggled those around flying times (the twins were six months). On holiday we hired a small minibus with a large back seat, and I made myself comfortable, and away we went.'*

MANY MOTHERS find that they are able to breastfeed whenever and wherever they need, without it ever becoming a problem. All you need is confidence, as these mothers testify.

Colette wonders whether her lack of embarrassment was related to her age – maturity gave her more confidence perhaps: *'In the Aberdeen area there are very few feeding facilities in public places, so Francis was fed in the car, in parks, in restaurants – wherever. I did not encounter any opposition to this; I even fed him during take-off on a flight to London, and on a BR train. I feel that most people would rather see a baby fed than hear it screaming its head off – I am sure that a few people (mostly men) did look the other way when they saw me plug Francis in, but I don't blame them for this as I know that it is sometimes difficult to know what to do in such a situation. So little public breastfeeding is seen these days that it isn't surprising (though certainly regrettable) that people are a bit fazed by it on occasions.'*

Louise and her husband thrive on the convenience of breastfeeding and Louise suggests: *'My one tip is not to ask if it's OK – the one time I asked if I could feed him I was told "No"! My husband and I also do a lot of walking, so breastfeeding is perfect. I've fed out on Saddleworth moor on numerous occasions!'*

Feeding in public came easily to Sheila: *'I fed Helen everywhere, standing in a car park, cafés, airports, on the bus, on a bench in the High Street. Always discreetly wearing lift-up T-shirts, not button up clothes. Sometimes I would be talking to someone who would suddenly realise I was feeding Helen. From seven months Helen would pull away too much for comfortable discretion. By then it wasn't a problem though as I would rarely be out for her few feeds.'*

More words of encouragement from Jillian: *'I would like to say to other mothers, don't be afraid to feed your baby in public as it can be done very discreetly; in fact go out as much as you can while your baby only needs milk as it gets much harder and messier whilst they are being weaned. I have fed in all sorts of places. I have never asked permission and I have never sat and fed in a "Mother's Room" or a loo as I don't think of feeding a baby as an activity to be hidden away. The reaction of other people (if any) has always been neutral or positive.'*

It's possible to feed your baby anywhere, as Moira proved: *'I can't remember ever thinking, "No, not in here". I wasn't a militant, determined to breastfeed to prove a point. I just never found myself in a situation where I couldn't feed my son discreetly, and so I simply fed him wherever I was. The only time I ever used any sort of special facility was in Mothercare or Boots when I was out shopping in the cold. In nice weather I've fed Francis outdoors – on a seat in a pedestrian precinct I was chatting to a friend all the time, and I don't think that anyone except me and her knew that I was nursing too. I've*

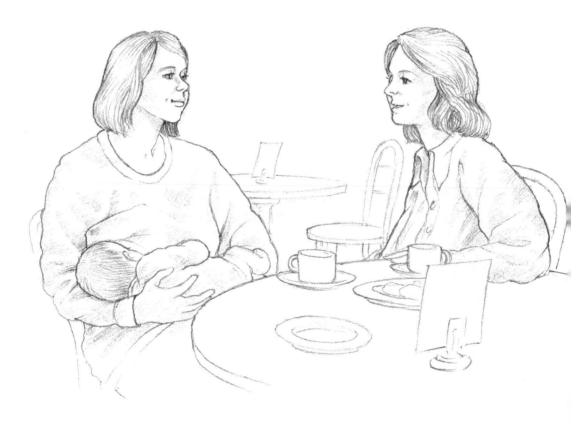

fed him in parks, on beaches, in restaurants at home and abroad, in the saloon of a cross-channel ferry, in pubs, on an aeroplane, in a wood. I've even fed him on more than one occasion while giving a lecture. I fed him on a hospital trolley while waiting for a scan. And I never felt, or was made to feel, uncomfortable doing it.'

THE REACTIONS of others to seeing women breastfeeding in public places can be interesting. Displaying breasts as sexual objects of desire and titillation is clearly quite acceptable: witness 'page three'. Meantime, we hear of a mother, quietly breastfeeding her baby, being asked to leave the local department store. Something is very strange indeed.

During a talk given at the 1995 NCT Annual Conference, Elizabeth Bradley, a child psychiatrist and psychoanalyst from the Tavistock Clinic in London, suggested that some people who express and display negative reactions to women breastfeeding their babies may do so as a result of a resurgence of their own latent and largely unconscious memories of an unsatisfactory breastfeeding relationship with their own mothers. Consequently, they may be almost completely out of touch with the needs of the baby for the comfort derived from his mother's breast. Conversely, those that feel comfortable seeing a baby at the breast are in touch with the needs of the baby and maybe have their own good memories of breastfeeding.

Is it fair that a breastfeeding woman should be burdened with the worries of other people's reactions to her feeding her baby? On one occasion, during a discussion at an antenatal class, it was suggested that there could be adverse reactions to a woman breastfeeding in public places. One young man stated quite categorically that other people's feelings were their business and their problem and not going to affect how he and his partner were going to feed their baby. Hopefully, his confidence carried them through to ensure a very positive breastfeeding experience.

A breastfed baby can be wonderfully 'transportable' since his nutritional requirements are readily available as long as he is not too far away from his mother.

Lois discovered just how easy it is to travel with a breastfed baby: *'I took my daughter along to several parties and social events and was able to breastfeed her on these occasions without attracting any adverse comments or looks. On one occasion one person did not even believe I was breastfeeding her as we were quite discreet and my daughter was so quiet and peaceful that he was convinced she was simply asleep in my arms.*

When my daughter was nine months old my partner and I took her on a four-week round the world trip. The fact that I was still breastfeeding her had several advantages. She became somewhat unsettled at times during the trip, due to frequently changing time zones and sleeping in numerous different cots and putting her to the breast was the most effective way of giving her comfort and a feeling of security. From a practical point of view, by breastfeeding, we did not have to worry about carrying formula milk around with us, sterilising bottles or finding sterile water. This trip certainly reinforced my belief in the positive effects of breastfeeding. I think many women are wary of breastfeeding in public and expect to meet hostility, which is a sad situation as if breastfeeding is to become more accepted as "normal" then its profile does need to be raised.'

For some women, like Brenda, although their confidence does grow as the baby grows, they never become completely happy breastfeeding 'just anywhere': *'Initially I only breastfed in front of men if they were family members or new fathers, but as time went by I learned to relax more in public. Before visiting cafés or art galleries I would check whether breastfeeding was permitted. I would use cloakrooms or empty rooms whenever possible.'*

ALTHOUGH THERE has been some increase in recent years in the provision of breastfeeding facilities in public places, there is still considerable room for improvement. Some public authorities, such as health and local authorities, are setting a positive example by making clear that breastfeeding is welcome on their premises.[47]

In order to encourage and support women to be able to breastfeed for as long as they wish, there needs to be a wider awareness of the value of the breastfeeding relationship and an increase in the facilities available in public places for the women who choose to breastfeed privately. A National Baby Care Symbol was launched in 1985 to encourage the provision of feeding and changing facilities in public places. If you see the symbol, you will find a mother and baby room which meets basic minimum standards of cleanliness, warmth, privacy, seating and hand-washing facilities.

Breastfeeding and sex

THE PUBLIC confusion of breasts for breastfeeding and breasts as sex objects may spill over into your personal relationship with your partner. The relationship you may have perhaps taken for granted has to be rethought. 'Does breastfeeding interfere with sex?' is a question many new parents ask.

Giving birth is an intensely physical and emotional experience and caring for a new baby is often all-engrossing. In so many ways being pregnant, giving birth and caring for a new baby is a disruption to your sexual relationship as a couple. No matter how many books you read or classes you attend, you cannot ever truly prepare for the changes that a baby brings. Living through this time, you will need to renegotiate your sexual relationship as a couple according to a constantly changing set of circumstances.

It may not be openly acknowledged in our society, but some men find their partners quite sexy when they are breastfeeding. This could be as a result of the increase in breast size or it may be some more deep-seated emotional satisfaction.

Lynn describes how her sexual relationship with her husband deepened: *'My husband found my breasts very sexy after the birth of our daughter – particularly my nipples. He found they were larger (or more prominent) as feeding had softened them, drawing them out. I also found my nipples more sensitive to stimulation and enjoyed them being touched when we made love – far more than before. I'd also lost some of my inhibitions about having my breasts touched during sex as I'd become more "at home" with my body whilst breastfeeding. Leaking milk became a joke rather than a cause for embarrassment and we were happy to use a towel under. I feel sharing the birth experience together and having my husband's support during breastfeeding enabled me to enjoy and share my body more with him when we made love. Tiredness and sleepless nights were far more detrimental to our sexual relationship than breastfeeding!'*

For some women, like Sharon, there is an overwhelming sense of change as a result of their experience of birth and mothering, which can bring new confidence: *'Before I breastfed, I was self-conscious of my breasts, my figure and weight and very absorbed in being a successful career woman who was as close to perfect as possible. Now, after breastfeeding I feel so womanly and okay with my weight and figure (even though I'm twenty pounds overweight still) and I feel confident in a way I never knew existed!'*

IN THE early months of a baby's life, it is quite possible that you will both be exhausted physically and emotionally and you may find that sleep becomes a much-needed commodity. It could be said that your sex drive is temporarily sublimated into other activities. Once you have begun to make love again after the birth, there may be other irritating difficulties to overcome together, as Colette relates: *'I frequently felt so engorged I couldn't bear my husband to touch me. I also found out very late on (baby about seven months) that breastfeeding tends to inhibit vaginal secretions presumably because it inhibits ovulation and production of oestrogen, making intercourse very sore and painful – until I realised this I was quite concerned about what could be wrong with me, and had visions of having been stitched up too tightly after birth or something. I wish the NCT had told me to anticipate this.'*

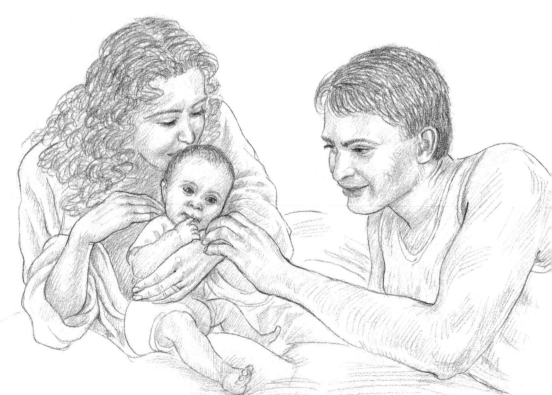

THE HORMONE responsible for initiating the let down of the milk from the breasts – oxytocin – is the hormone involved in orgasm, so you could breastfeed the baby before making love to avoid a shower of milk interrupting proceedings.

Or do as Linda did: *'Sex was more fulfilling after birth for both of us, though my husband kept clear of my breasts until approximately twelve months after the birth, which although I was still breastfeeding, was when my breasts stopped leaking. Wearing a bra with pads in helped prevent interruptions of leaking milk during breast stimulation by my husband.'*

IF YOU both can share your positive and negative feelings, there is a far greater chance of your relationship remaining healthy and emotionally nourishing for you both. Sadly, sometimes the arrival of a baby may bring some real worries about your relationship to the surface. In these circumstances it would be wise to seek expert help to enable you to talk through your concerns together.

Most couples will be able to work together to ensure their sexual relationship continues. Hopefully you will enjoy doing so; perhaps you may also explore new areas of stimulation and enjoyment of each other at this time.

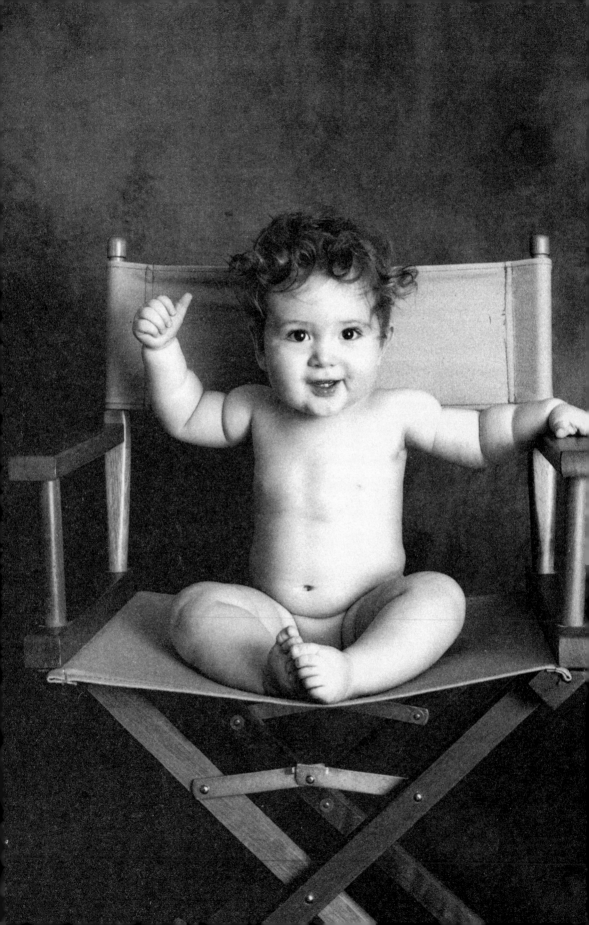

CHAPTER **six** *Moving towards independence*

AT AROUND six months (younger in some babies, older in others), you will begin to introduce food other than breast milk to your baby. It is a new experience for him and represents a movement away from the very secure, natural and comforting activity of being held and cradled in his mother's arms while feeding.

INTRODUCING OTHER FOOD

INTRODUCING OTHER foods ends the total dependency that your baby has on you. Women react differently to this. Some are pleased to arrive at this stage, others are sad to see their baby taking his first moves away from them. Interestingly, some second-time mothers may delay introducing other foods, as they do not want to encourage the baby to grow up too soon, nor to cope with the extra chores involved.

His first reactions may not be too positive. Instead of the pleasure of a warm, malleable breast, your baby must get used to the feel of a hard, possibly cold spoon, first touching his lips and then later being placed in his mouth. The watchword is to go gently and gradually. There is no rush; breast milk will be the most valuable food for him for quite some time.

Irene started her baby on solids gradually at about four and a half months and there were no major problems: *'Life seems to get better and better. By the time she was eating three meals a day, she was still feeding from the breast six to eight times a day. This slowly dwindled to four to six times a day by the time she was a year old and later to three to four times a day.'*

It was a similar initial experience for Sandy and her baby: *'I started to wean Linda at about five months. This was a very gradual process; she took solids very well. As she had more solids, she gradually cut out her breastfeeds.*

It seemed a very natural process which she would dictate. At one year Linda was having a breastfeed on waking and one before bed.'

YOUR NEW baby is not capable of digesting complex food substances. The Department of Health recommends exclusive breastfeeding for at least the first four months of life. For potentially allergic babies, it is better to wait until they are around six months if possible before introducing solids. A baby's capacity to digest and so utilise other foods is determined by the maturity of his gut; that is, by his age not by his weight or the length of time he sleeps. As his gut matures, different enzymes are produced which enable him to digest other substances as well as milk. However, whilst he is developing, during the first two years of life, breast milk continues to be the easiest source of food for your baby, from which he derives a high nutritional benefit.

Initially offering other foods can be as low key as possible. The idea is to offer the baby an opportunity to try new tastes and a slightly different texture. Many mothers begin by introducing baby rice mixed with breast milk. The familiar smell of your breast milk may be reassuring for your baby. Introducing one new taste at a time is beneficial and your baby's reaction can be watched, particularly if there is a history of food intolerances in the family.

'I was still feeding a number of times at night so this time (a second baby) I introduced solids in the hope that she might sleep longer. Although she loved the solids it made no difference to the number of breastfeeds she had.'

THIS WAS Debbie's experience and like many mothers she had heard that introducing solid food will ensure a baby will sleep for longer periods at night or automatically reduce the times he breastfeeds. Considering the quantities involved in the early stages of weaning, this seems unlikely. Since a baby's digestive system is not capable of fully digesting more complex foods until he is older, the quantity of milk he receives remains important. Sometimes a baby may even wake more frequently in order to ensure he receives his necessary milk, like Joe, Dawn's baby, did: *'When Joe was about nine weeks old, he became difficult to satisfy. Since by this time, he weighed 15lb, I suggested to Val (my health visitor) that I should start to introduce solids. I knew that this was rather earlier than the accepted three to four months, but Joe was distinctly heavier than was expected for babies of his age. To begin with, I was very careful what I gave Joe. He started with baby rice, mixed with expressed breast milk, followed by a variety of puréed fruits and vegetables. He soon showed a liking for stronger flavours; by the time he was six months, he was eating breakfast, lunch and dinner. He was still feeding from me first thing in the morning, mid-morning, mid-afternoon and at bedtime, but then he slept through until morning.'*

FEEDING FILE

Tips for introducing other foods

● Try not to be influenced too much by what other babies are doing, their eating or sleeping patterns

● If your baby is less than four months try increasing the milk feeds he receives before introducing other foods

● Offer his first tastes after his usual breastfeed

● Sometime after introducing solids to your baby he may accept a 'breast sandwich': that is – one breast, solids, other breast

● Start at an unhurried time of the day

● Hold the baby on your knee for the first tastes

● Use a flattish, small, sturdy plastic spoon. Place it on the baby's lips and let him 'lap' his first tastes

● Simple puréed fruits may be easy starter foods

● If he doesn't like it, leave it a few days and try again

● Use packets or jars if it is easier for you to avoid the feeling of him rejecting your own prepared food

● Read the labels, so you know what he is receiving

● If he has had enough, let him tell you. Don't force it

● Offer a fairly wide selection of tastes, he may like what you do not

● If he is off-colour he may not accept other foods, go back to fully breastfeeding for the time being

● Breast milk is a good base for a mixed diet – as long as your baby is taking plenty of milk you can take weaning on to solids at a more leisurely pace

● Some NCT breastfeeding counsellors offer weaning classes. Ask the local branch

● For more information on *Your baby's first vegetables* read the leaflet produced by the National Childbirth Trust and the National Farmers' Union. Available from the National Farmers' Union, 164 Shaftesbury Avenue, London. Tel. 0171 331 7200.

A YOUNG BABY will associate the satisfaction of his hunger pangs with suckling. When he cries from hunger he will come to expect to suck. In the early stages of weaning, then, it may be most useful to offer the usual breastfeed first and then offer a taste of the new food. Holding your baby in your arms will be reassuring, and using a fairly flat, sturdy plastic spoon will also help things go smoothly. The consistency of the first foods is very 'runny' and your baby can 'lap' from a flat spoon when it is placed to his lips. Good, gentle experiences for your baby will set the scene for later feeding. As time passes, your baby will accept greater quantities and a wide range of tastes and textures.

When Elaine's baby, David, was three months old she introduced solids into his diet in the form of baby rice, mixed with some of her expressed breast milk: *'I also gave him gluten free, low sugar Liga rusks which I softened with a little boiled water then added a little of my expressed milk to give him the familiar taste and smell. He would eat this with no hesitation whatsoever, and sometimes wanted more! I would follow with a breastfeed. He took to solids well and by four months was having breakfast, lunch and tea followed by a breastfeed.'*

SOME WOMEN do not find it easy to introduce other foods to their baby. There is no doubt that there will be more washing-up, more messy clothes, and smellier nappies to deal with. There is also the decision about what to give a baby at this stage. Labels like 'sugar free', 'gluten free' or 'best for baby' or 'fortified with' or 'additional factor X' all seem to have resulted in confusion for parents. There is a multi-million-pound industry surrounding the manufacture and marketing of baby foods. Potent advertising could lead to you believing that a particular food is necessary for your baby or, even worse, that it is somehow superior to what can be produced easily and simply in the kitchen. There is no money for the manufacturer if you buy a fresh apple and prepare your own puréed apple for your baby.

If your baby does not like a taste he is likely to either close his mouth or let it dribble out of his mouth. If you have spent some time preparing a special food for your baby, you may find it difficult to accept his reaction; perhaps feel a bit rejected. It is very tempting to go on offering the food. Ready-prepared foods are very valuable here. It is much easier to throw away food that has come from a packet.

This all comes from food being associated with love. Try to be aware of your feelings and avoid getting too emotionally involved with the food you are offering. Some women continue exclusive breastfeeding until they and their babies are ready to start solids. There is evidence that exclusive breastfeeding for at least the first 13 weeks confers numerous health benefits on the baby.[48]

BREASTFEEDING THE OLDER BABY

BREASTFEEDING AN older baby is a special experience. Each baby has a unique personality and there is a lot to enjoy together, as Patti describes: *'A high point I will always remember was the time when my 14-month-old daughter sucked twice to get the let down started, then cheekily looked up at me, smiled then disappeared below my jumper only to blow a "raspberry" on my tummy as a joke. She, of course, was back latched on in time to catch the rush of milk.'*

For Lesley, the pleasure of breastfeeding has increased with time: *'Eleven months later, the milk is still on tap and we both enjoy the closeness and reassurance that feeding gives. I keep intending to cut Mary's feeds down to two a day – first thing in the morning and last thing at night – but we cannot cut down the cuddles and 'snacks' in between – well, there's not much of a problem with that – breastfeeding won't last for ever, and really we're both making the most of it while we can – and what's wrong with that?'*

CHOOSING TO carry on breastfeeding may mean that you will be exposed to comments and criticism. The attitudes of others are not always encouraging. There seems to be an unwritten law that some people would like recognised: breastfeeding is all right, but not in public or when the baby is older. The query then, of course, is what constitutes an 'older baby'. There could be as many suggestions as there are people willing to voice them. Common ones are: not when the baby can eat other food, not once he has teeth, or can wear shoes or walk about.

Some families seem to raise the issue that breastfeeding a baby beyond an unspecified age could lead to something sexual. Often, sexual matters will not be discussed openly in families and consequently any disapproval might be expressed as innuendo. Where explanations have been forthcoming, the following have been offered to some women. For example: breastfeeding a boy child too long could mean that he becomes too fixated on his mother, or develops too great an interest in women's breasts as an adult. Breastfeeding a girl child beyond a certain age may reduce her capacity to relate effectively to men. There is no evidence for any of these tales.

Vanessa describes how amazed she was when she came across this type of prejudice in her own family: *'One of my father's cousins breastfed her little boy until he was about four and I remember family rumblings about this. Looking back, I think two factors influenced their thinking: firstly, that she was in some way "spoiling" the boy, indulging him, not asserting her own will by "allowing" him to continue to have access to her whenever he liked; secondly, a concern regarding sexuality, that she might be deriving some sensual pleasure from this form of contact. Nature has designed breastfeeding species – why deny its sensuality? It seems that there is often more concern when the child still breastfeeding is a boy!'*

SOMETIMES OBJECTIONS are also put forward that breastfeeding will be detrimental to your physical health and you will become too dependent upon your child for emotional satisfaction. Again, there is no evidence to support this.

Hearing these sorts of comments or just being aware that something is disapproved of can lead to a lot of soul searching and sometimes you may begin to feel you must justify what you are doing. You may have to be quite assertive or develop an 'impermeable' layer, as Amy discovered with her third baby when he was eighteen months old: *'The other day someone asked me, "What is it like to feed a toddler who is walking around?" All I could think to say was that it wasn't at all strange and I found myself saying, "Well, it isn't like feeding a toddler, I am feeding Robert, just as I have since he was born." In thinking over this incident later my reply reminded me of the ongoing nature of the feeding relationship, that it is very much a two-way thing that is not strictly under your control as it involves another party. With my third child I had no preconceived ideas about when I was likely to wean him and was inclined to trust my own instincts rather than seeking outside opinions.'*

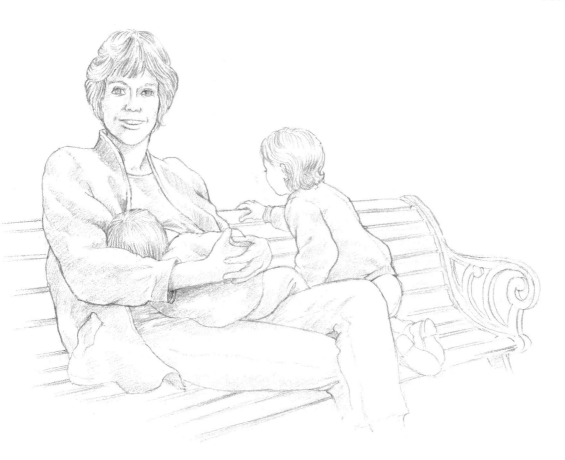

Sunita also experienced critical comments: *'Outside of the home I felt very aware of embarrassment whilst nursing a toddler – even before she was a year old people would remark on her still being "attached". I also encountered some hostility when I took her to a local Tweeny Tumbler session – feeling slightly at odds, Jane asked to nurse. Once attached, I was then informed that no food or drink was allowed. I really cannot view breastfeeding as being in the same category as all other forms of food and stalked off feeling humiliated and embarrassed.'*

YOU MAY not make a definite decision to continue breastfeeding, but if everything is comfortable between you and your baby, breastfeeding just becomes part of the day-to-day life you share. In fact, breastfeeding may have become quite an insignificant part of life you share together. The focus for other people may be rather different.

Irene fed her baby for more than nineteen months, but found the social pressures were getting stronger: *'I found that situation hard to cope with. I didn't think I was flaunting it and very rarely did she feed unless we were at home (except if we were at a friend's at nap time). She didn't ask for it when we were out and about, and I felt, despite some pretty heavy comments, good about it. Unfortunately from the people I spoke to, I gained the feeling that: What was I doing still feeding at nineteen months? Wasn't there a detrimental affect to myself? The people who did support "longer" feeding were wonderful and really did make me feel much better about the "Should I?" and "Why?" but on the whole I found the majority of people unbelievably insensitive.'*

Sunita firmly believes that breastfeeding becomes more useful as your baby grows older: *'To me it seemed natural to carry on with something that worked so well, which calms an emotional toddler so easily and sends her off to sleep in a matter of minutes. Toddlers rarely understand their own emotions and can't really cope with them either. Neither can we as adults cope with our toddlers at times – breastfeeding calms both them and us so easily.'*

SOME WOMEN decide to handle and counter negative comments by gaining more information, making a very positive choice to continue breastfeeding their babies. Others, like Paula, acknowledge the benefits of longer breastfeeding and clearly appreciate the closeness that breastfeeding provides in all sorts of situations: *'As I write this, Charlotte is now fourteen months old and I feel no urgency to be done with breastfeeding. I believe that breast milk continues to be of importance during the second year of life. There are times such as when she may be off-colour and she will refuse solid foods, I am able to offer her the breast which is a great comfort to her. Breast milk is easily digested and nourishing for a feverish baby too. I feel a special closeness with her when she is poorly and I am thankful that I can respond to her in such an intimate, physical way.*

On a more day-to-day level, Charlotte has turned out to be a fussy eater. Her diet consists largely of peanut butter sandwiches and garlic bread. She refuses all fruit and vegetables (potatoes and roast parsnips excepted). I consider that breast milk makes an important contribution to her restricted diet – in fact, it is probably her only decent source of vitamins!

I think that breast milk forms a solid back-up against the vagaries of ill health and faddy eating. It is, if you like, my insurance policy. I have found breastfeeding for me creates a perfect way to respond to my baby with passion, tenderness, comfort and, of course, love.'

Vanessa and her partner both acknowledge the special bond of breast-feeding: *'I am now aware that there* are *physiological benefits in breastfeeding the older baby (Rachel will soon be two); I am still passing antibodies to her through my milk. I am also reassured that the psychological benefits, to both of us, are immeasurable – she can find comfort from my breast and I am able to give this in a unique and loving way.*

I particularly enjoy our feeds before bedtime – it is a quiet, private and peaceful time for both of us and I love the fact that she can not only communicate her desire for "Mummy milk" but she can acknowledge her enjoyment of it – in reply to my asking if it's nice she nods her head vigorously. Although breastfeeding gives Rachel and me a special relationship, it is quite an exclusive one. My husband and I have had to acknowledge that and talk about this, as at times it has meant totally separate bedtime routines for us and our children. Without his understanding and support it would have been difficult to carry on.

I am pleased that my breastfeeding journey with Rachel has gone so well, particularly as she is a girl. It seems important to me; I suppose it's because I hope that one day she will be able to experience for herself those same feelings of joy that I felt whilst feeding her. I must admit to being a "closet" breast-feeder now. Whilst Rachel was still a baby, i.e. crawling and gurgling, I felt at ease breastfeeding in public. Now I feel less inclined. For one thing I have reverted back to wearing normal, under-wired bras which make access to my breasts less easy. It is harder to be discreet when feeding a toddler, Rachel tends to pull my clothing about and wants to play with my other nipple whilst feeding! I still do not feel ready to give up this precious, privileged, mutually enjoyable and satisfying process. I know it must come one day; I suppose it will happen gradually and maybe I won't realise that the last breastfeed has happened.'

Feeding a toddler can be amusing at times, as Fiona, mother of three-year-old Penny, describes: *'There is a social joy in feeding an older child which you don't get with a baby. Every morning we walked with Sarah, my older daughter, to her nursery school and when we got home Penny would say, "Shall we have a nice drink, Mummy? Put the kettle on." She often commented if it was a particularly nice taste and once correctly guessed that I must have eaten some pineapples! One day she said that it was so nice today that she'd try the other side – would it be the same?*

I never suffered the difficulties that many women describe when feeding older children who "demand" it at inconvenient times and use words which the mother finds embarrassing at the supermarket checkout. Between us we sorted out without discussing it that Penny had her "nice drink" at certain times when we could both sit down and enjoy it. She only used to breastfeed for comfort when she was ill.'

Breastfeeding can be very useful during times of illness, as Joy found with her baby Flora: *'My youngest daughter Flora was breastfed until just before her third birthday. She stopped when she decided she didn't need a breastfeed at night. When she was about eighteen months old Flora had a horrible time with chickenpox; she was covered in spots, even her mouth and the back of her throat were swollen and spotty. She refused to put a beaker or cup in her mouth as it was too sore. I was relieved to be able to return to fully breastfeeding her for a few days. Like her sisters she has a tendency to wheezy, croupy colds, and I found letting her feed at night when she could have longer, comfort sucking, much more effective, and less exhausting for both of us, than spending the night in a steamy bathroom.'*

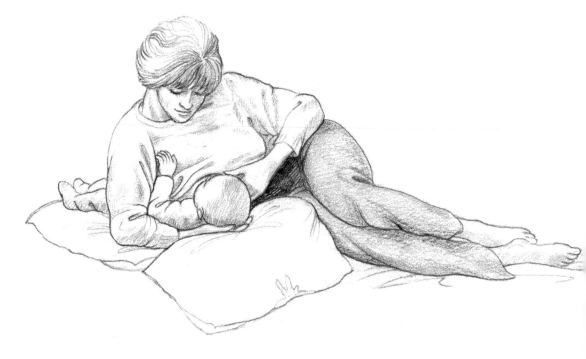

Leigh knows that her daughter Emily relishes her 'mummy milk' and for her too it has been a time of great self-awareness: *'I have enjoyed the closeness it has brought in all the different stages of Emily's development from baby to pre-school child. It has been a handy soother and the ultimate fast-food snack. This way gradually stopping is giving each of us a chance to find other ways of being close and expressing our love. I feel a tremendous bond with my daughter and feel that this is in part because of our long breastfeeding relationship.'*

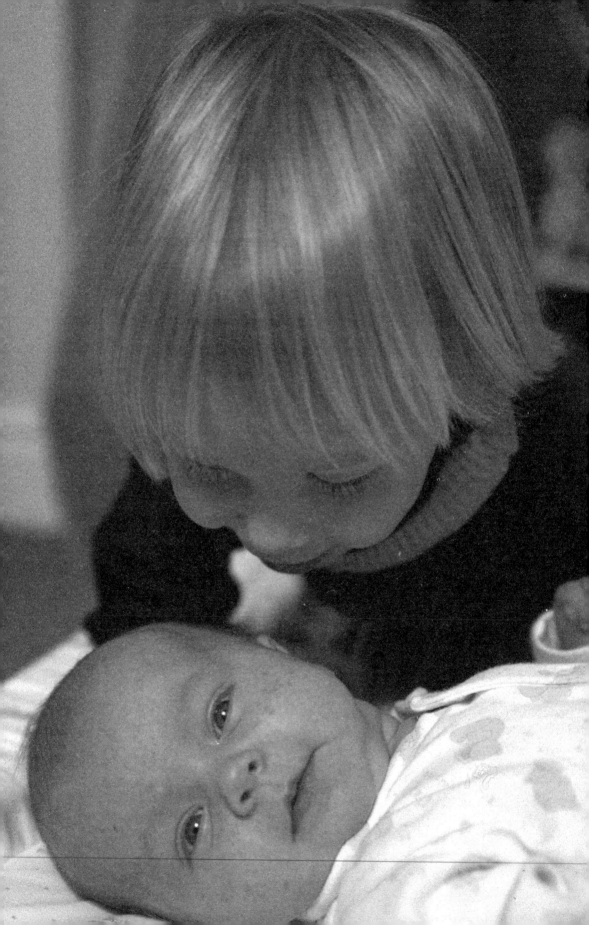

CHAPTER ***seven*** *A*
breastfeeding
family

ANOTHER BABY?

IT MAY BE an effort for you as a mother of one child to take the time
to prepare yourself physically and emotionally for the next birth.
Attending antenatal classes may not be so easy when there are other
children to consider. If you do arrange care for your older child and
attend NHS antenatal classes or NCT refresher courses, you will find
it is a real pleasure to focus on yourself and the new baby. Time to
think about how it will be to have another baby to care for as well,
both the practical and emotional aspects, is all important, as is time to
enjoy thinking about your coming baby.

Practical aspects, such as: 'Where will the new baby sleep?'; 'How
will we all fit in the car?'; 'What will happen to the toddler whilst I'm
in labour?'; 'Will there be sufficient money coming in?' may all feature as concerns.

Emotional aspects usually centre on worries about coping with the
demands of the first child whilst coping with the demands of a new
baby: 'Can there be enough hours in the day?'; 'How will it feel to
relate to two or maybe three little children?'; 'Who do you feed
first?'; 'How will the older child behave?'; 'Whose needs come first?'
There are so many questions to consider.

Perhaps the underlying question to many of these worries is: 'How
can it be possible to love another child as much as I love this one?'
Even if there has been a difficult start with the first baby and the path
of parenthood has been bumpy, most men and women fall hopelessly in love with their children. There is nothing so wonderful for a
parent as having a small trusting hand clutched in yours or to feel the
unconditional love which we might receive from our children. These
are truly very special experiences. Presumably some of this 'reward'
explains why many couples choose to have more than one child.

FEEDING FILE

THINKING ABOUT ANOTHER BABY AND BREASTFEEDING

Before the baby arrives

● Try to spend time talking with your older child about the arrival of another baby

● Photographs of him as a baby will show him how helpless he once was

● Photographs of him breastfeeding or meeting other breastfed babies would help to familiarise him with breastfeeding

● Do not expect him to share your joy at the prospect of another baby or tell him how lucky he will be to have a playmate. New babies are not good at playing anything

● If your toddler still has a daytime sleep, try to preserve it. That short time during the afternoon will be really valuable for you after the baby arrives

● If possible, do not schedule any major changes to coincide with the arrival of the new baby. For example, getting used to having a new baby brother or sister is enough to handle without starting playschool or nursery as well

● It might be possible to get a dolly and cradle for your older child so that he could care for 'his' baby as you care for the new arrival

● There may be picture books at the library that could lead to chats about what life might be like. For example: 'Sometimes Daddy will get the breakfast. Mummy will have to breastfeed quite a lot'

● If your toddler is of that age, delay potty training until well after the new baby arrives

● Encourage him to sit with you as you rest towards the end of pregnancy. There will be times when you are feeding the new baby when your older child could sit with you as you feed. When you are breastfeeding, you will have an arm free to cuddle him

● Choose a box of toys that will only be brought out when you're breastfeeding. Let your toddler choose which toys go in that box and maybe give it a special name, so that he knows both the box of toys and breastfeeding are special.

Some forward planning about coping with two (or more) children is valuable, but much of the future as a family is really a 'wait and see' situation. Perhaps it is reassuring to say that most parents find that the 'quantity' of love available grows with each additional child. It is not a case of having to divide the 'quantity' of love by the number of children.

FEEDING FILE

THINKING ABOUT ANOTHER BABY AND BREASTFEEDING

After the baby is born

● The new baby is a competitor for your attention. Moving him on from being the baby to the 'big boy' in the family is quite a challenge. Be prepared to be patient

● Try to think ahead and have a drink, a book or toys ready for your older child before you start to breastfeed the new baby

● It is a worthwhile investment to spend time with your older child when the new baby sleeps. Resist the temptation to dash around doing the household chores. Your older child is your baby too and he will need a lot of reassurance that you still love him. Spending time with him is the best assurance you can offer

● Your older child may ask to try out your breast milk. He may even remember breastfeeding himself. Try to accept his request. Go through the motions of offering him your breast. The probability is that he will not remember how to suckle and he will lose interest. Those youngsters who can suckle usually do not like the taste of the breast milk. Allowing his natural curiosity is most likely to result in his interest passing on to something else

● Talk to your older child, tell him how you feel, ask him how he feels. He will under-

stand much more than you might realise and pick up on your tensions. Maybe by talking, you will be able to maintain a relaxed atmosphere. It is certainly worth a try

● Life will be rather hectic as you adjust to caring for more than one child, but it does become easier

● Your older child does not need a very busy social life at this time. He needs you in a reasonable state of mind much more. Invest in plenty of home activities for the older child, such as play-dough, sticking, construction toys. Cut out all but essential trips and reserve your energies, just for the time being

● Enlist the help of well-known relatives and friends. A short time spent away from you and the new baby may ease any tension that develops

● Some community centres organise parent, baby and toddler groups

● Local National Childbirth Trust branches organise get-togethers where you could breastfeed in a friendly atmosphere while the older children play together. Chatting with other mothers is always valuable.

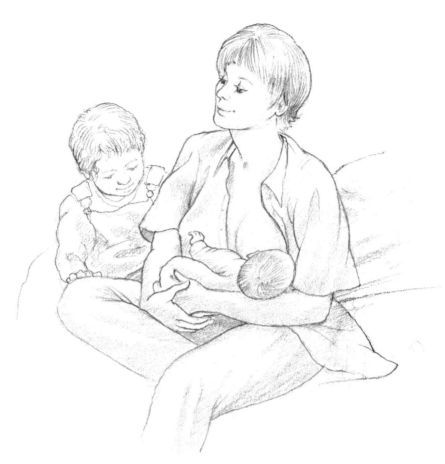

TANDEM FEEDING

QUITE A FEW women cease breastfeeding in order to encourage their menstrual cycle to return to normal so that they may conceive another baby. It is possible that you may become pregnant while you are still breastfeeding your baby or toddler. Some older babies naturally 'go off' the breast milk at this point, as it seems that the taste may change, due to the changing hormones in your bloodstream. Your nipples may become quite sensitive during the early stages of pregnancy and you may consciously or unconsciously encourage your baby or toddler to stop breastfeeding.

Anna fed her first baby until she was three: *'She loved feeding and I loved feeding her. Gradually she fed less, as other things became important to her. She stopped when I became pregnant. Perhaps the milk tasted different or* there wasn't as much of it. She wasn't upset about it, she just didn't want to feed any more.'

IF THE early stages of your next pregnancy pass without your older child stopping breastfeeding, you may find yourself contemplating breastfeeding both the new baby and your toddler – tandem feeding.

This may not always be an easy experience, as Dawn explains: '*I breastfed my first child for two years and three months and in fact was still feeding her whilst in labour with my son. Once feeding was established my son was voracious and doubled his birth weight at nine weeks. I tried to feed both children, but my supply matched my toddler's demands. I quickly became exhausted and my midwife said I must stop feeding my toddler immediately, and explained to my daughter why she couldn't have "milkies" any more.*

I now know that I should have made greater efforts prior to the baby's birth to wean her, as the whole episode has been very painful and traumatic for both of us.'

Dawn had a mixed experience: whilst she continued breastfeeding during pregnancy, she seemed to be responding to the needs of her toddler, but once the baby was born the situation became more complex.

Morag found that she really enjoyed tandem feeding: '*My eldest child, nearly three, was still breastfeeding when her sister was born. It was a really special feeling to have both of my children cuddled up to me, breastfeeding together. Before her sister was born, the eldest was only breastfeeding three or four times a day, but for the first month or so afterwards she wanted to do so every time the baby did. That made life a lot easier for me: no trying to amuse a bored and jealous toddler whilst breastfeeding the new baby, just a chance to sit and relax together. I was confident that my body would respond to the extra suckling, and it did. I had masses of milk, so never had worries as to whether the baby would get enough.'*

If you are in this situation, it is valuable to allow your new baby free and first access to your breasts in the early weeks. This ensures that the new baby receives the vital colostrum and has the opportunity to build up his own milk supply.

ANXIETIES

FOR SOME women a second pregnancy may bring very real anxieties about feeding; Sophie explains: *'"Pregnant", I heard myself saying, "how wonderful". A baby brother or sister for my five-year-old son Paul. The initial excitement of the news wore off when I remembered the dreadful experience I had had with breastfeeding Paul. The first six weeks of my son's life, spent trying to force my breasts upon him, the pain, the tears and the frustration! Well not this time – I was in control with this baby. I'd already been there, done that and failed miserably! What was the point of putting myself and my new baby through all that, when I knew perfectly well that breastfeeding was not for me? No, the decision had been made, no breastfeeding this baby – bottles here we come! Having made the decision I sat back and enjoyed the next nine months, everything clear in my head about my preferred method of feeding.'*

Martha is expecting her second baby soon and plans to bottle-feed from the start: *'Although I appreciate that there were many reasons why I rejected my daughter I am absolutely convinced that breastfeeding played a major part in my unhappiness and depression. I am equally certain that things will be better this time, now the burden of guilt of not breastfeeding has been lifted.'*

Rebecca is pregnant again: *'This time I have an open mind. If breastfeeding works, well then I will breastfeed. If it doesn't, I will bottle-feed. I would like to know what it is like to suckle a baby, I would like to give my baby the best food possible, and I would like to avoid the expense and hassle of buying and preparing formula milk, but if breastfeeding doesn't work out, I do know that bottle-feeding is not the end of the world.'*

IN MOST cases, second and subsequent babies are generally delivered more easily and breastfeeding is established in a relaxed and gentle way. The 1990 *Infant Feeding* survey[1] found that women were more likely to breastfeed the second baby if they had breastfed the first.

This was certainly the case for Vanessa: *'With Rachel, my second baby, the birth experience was much different. She was born into water in a quiet and dimly lit room and was put to my breast within the first hour of her life and sucked for a little while. She slept a lot that day but towards the evening woke and had her first "real" feed. I felt confident enough to try feeding her lying down in the hospital bed (something I never mastered the first time). The hospital staff left me alone – they could see I was fine.'*

Tanya also found the second time around easier: *'I had no real problems when my second child was born at home eleven months ago. I still found the first few days a bit unnerving, waiting for my milk supply to establish and we got to know each other.'*

Carly had had a bad breastfeeding experience the first time: *'But this time it was different. My baby did settle and she slept. I believed in myself and I knew this time what I had to offer was the very best. No one could diffuse my nurturing instinct.'*

IF YOU have had a difficult breastfeeding experience with your first baby, you may need to come to terms with a lot of mixed feelings. There may be a sense of your body letting you down in some way; you may wonder why breastfeeding was so difficult for you when it is supposed to be a natural process. You might also wonder if it is worth trying again. There could be the possibility that it will not go well and so there could be further disappointment. Some women cope with these feelings of disappointment at the time, crying and expressing their feelings to those around them. Gradually they may be able to put the experience behind them. However, there are some women who will have dealt with their disappointment by burying it, not talking about it or discussing it. If you are in this situation, it is possible that the fears you have about breastfeeding will surface as the expected date of delivery of the next baby draws nearer. In these circumstances, it is really important that you try to talk through your worries, per-haps with your midwife or an NCT breastfeeding counsellor.

It does take courage to try again; many women have their courage rewarded the second or third time around, like Lorna: *'Delivery of one baby girl in July 1994, safe and sound, bring in the bottles I heard myself say. My husband wanted me to at least try to breastfeed so reluctantly I attempted to latch Carol on to my breast – thinking that I'll show him, I'll have a go, fail miserably like last time and he'll feel guilty and let me bottle-feed after all. WRONG! Carol latched on to my breast – sucked away happily and has done so contentedly ever since — no engorgement, no cracked nipples, no pain. Just one very happy baby. I still cannot believe it now six months on. I hated breast-feeding, it was the worst experience of my life, and yet with my second baby I have loved every minute of it. I'm so glad that my husband encouraged me to try again. I wouldn't have missed breastfeeding my daughter for the world.'*

Sandra's determination eventually rewarded her: *'It has taken me three attempts and three babies to achieve successful breastfeeding and now having fed Joel for six months I know there will be no bottles for him. No, this time breast is best. I am proud to have overcome my problems.'*

Gail defied her family's scepticism and with the arrival of her third child, she resolutely decided to try breastfeeding once more: *'This time I decided to ask for help from anyone who could. I met a breastfeeding counsellor during my pregnancy and told her of my previous problems and how*

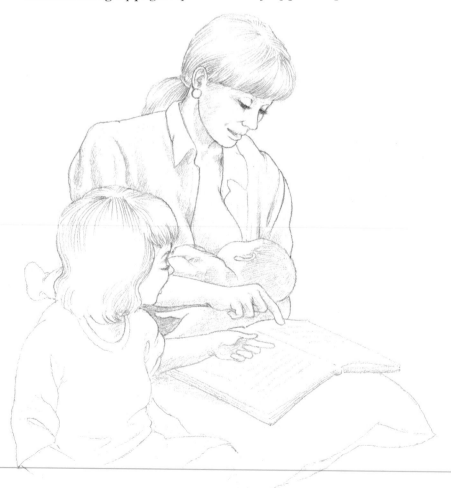

I still wanted to overcome them. By the time I got home with Arron (day four) I was fairly confident. I was soon hitching my T-shirt up in a professional manner whenever he opened his mouth. As a successful breastfeeder (at last) there is a wonderful feeling of fulfilment. Best of all, our two girls are seeing their mother breastfeed, and I hope it will serve them well in the future.'

OF COURSE, breastfeeding a second or third child means that there is a toddler or older child to care for as well. Many women meet together, sometimes in each other's homes, during the early days with a second or subsequent baby. The older children have company whilst their mothers chat and offer each other support. Also, by breastfeeding, at least there will be one arm and hand free to give affection to the other child, as Jinny and Laura discovered: *'I loved the convenience, especially as I now had a toddler I was trying to keep track of as well. It became our special quiet time. I would nurse and Jacob would curl up on the other side with a book or a puzzle, and we would read or sing songs to the baby. And having a toddler, breastfeeding was my time to really concentrate on the baby, the eye-to-eye and skin-to-skin contact especially when my husband was home and could entertain the toddler. I was much more active the second time; more errands to run, more places to be or take Jacob to. And I found the convenience of nursing invaluable.'*

'Some of my happiest memories of that time are sitting down in the cool of our lounge feeding the baby with my arm around his sister reading her a story. I asked myself then, and I still do now, how could I have coped with holding a baby and feeding him whilst holding a book and turning the pages if I'd been bottle-feeding?'

Morag found herself a source of entertainment: *'When my third daughter was born the eldest was nearly six and able to understand when I breastfed the two younger children. Sometimes she joined me on the sofa and "breastfed" her doll too!'*

BREASTFEEDING TWINS OR MORE

SOME COUPLES discover, during the pregnancy, that they are to be the parents of two babies. The dilemmas usually faced by parents of children that are born one at a time come all at once to the parents of

FEEDING FILE

BREASTFEEDING TWINS OR MORE

Individually or both at once?

The first decision you will be faced with is 'one at a time' or 'both together'? Anecdotal evidence suggests that feeding one baby at a time at first can help you to overcome individual difficulties with that baby, and may help you to begin an individual relationship with each of your babies. Simultaneous feeding becomes easier as the babies get older and more practised at latching on. However, simultaneous feeding provides greater stimulation to the milk supply, so this may be useful to build up a good initial supply. If you have help, you may choose to feed both together for this reason.

Positions for feeding

When it comes to bringing the babies together to the breast, there are several variations on a theme. The '**football hold**' is a good position for newborn twins. The babies are placed so that their body and legs are tucked under your arms, and their heads and necks are supported in your hands. The babies are held so that they are tucked in to your sides, with their tummies facing you. Pillows are used to give additional support, so that you are not bending over the babies. As the babies gain control of their heads, you will not need to support their heads, which leaves your arms free to hold a drink or read a book.

In the '**parallel hold**', one of the babies is held in the 'conventional' nursing position, across your body, and the other is held in the 'football' hold, so that the babies are lying parallel with each other, facing the same direction. Again, pillows will be needed to support the babies so that you are not supporting any weight. The babies should be held so that their tummies are facing you.

It is possible to hold both babies in the conventional nursing position, with one baby lying across the other. This is called the '**crisscross hold**'. It is important to check that both babies are in the correct position, with their bodies facing you.

There are no rules for positioning twins, other than the normal rules for good positioning. Each mother will discover for herself which position suits her best, and you may find that your babies have their own preferences too.

Choosing a breast

Some mothers choose to swap their babies to the other breast at each feed. Others prefer to keep one breast for each baby. Swapping breasts regularly will ensure that an even supply is maintained. This will help if one baby is noticeably stronger than the other, as the strong suckler will stimulate the supply for the weaker. However, keeping each baby to his own breast may be better for establishing that baby's milk supply to suit him, and will ensure that he gets sufficient hindmilk for growth. Some babies may develop a preference for one breast. Again, this is something which you will discover for yourself as your babies grow.

twins or more. An instant family: double trouble or twice the pleasure? Discovering that you are expecting twins – or more – may mean that you wonder if you can feed them both yourself. Often, women have little confidence that their bodies can produce enough milk for one baby, so when there are two babies, many mothers are led to believe that it will not be possible to fully breastfeed them both. In the past, women have always been able to feed more than one baby. Wet nurses commonly took on four to six babies at once.[49]

> ### Further help with twins or more
>
> Twins and Multiple Births Association (TAMBA), PO Box 30, Little Sutton, South Wirrel L66 1TH. Tel: 0151 348 0020. TAMBA provides a listening and information service on 01732 868000: Monday-Friday 6pm-11pm; Saturday and Sunday 10am-11pm. Your call will be answered by someone who is a parent of twins or more themselves. They also provide some useful leaflets on *Twins, Breastfeeding Twins* and *Bottle-feeding Twins*.

The principles of demand and supply still operate: if two babies are breastfeeding, your breasts will produce enough for two. A study in 1977 found that the prolactin response in women who are breastfeeding twins may be double that of mothers feeding only one baby.[50]

If you have already breastfed a baby, you are more likely to view the prospect of feeding more than one with optimism. You may find that other people – even the health professionals caring for you – are sceptical about your ability to breastfeed more than one baby. If you are able to talk to someone who is already breastfeeding twins, or if you have supportive carers, you can approach the prospect with anticipation rather than dread.

For Simone, the reality was even more complex – three babies!: '*After recovering from the shock of expecting triplets, and having staggered through the horrendous first few months of pregnancy, I eventually contacted other triplet parents to discuss the "terms and conditions" of a multiple birth. I discussed the feasibility of breastfeeding triplets with several families, and had accepted that our babies would have to be breast and bottle-fed if we were to survive. We had also accepted that our babies would probably spend several weeks in a special care baby unit, and therefore I would need to use a breast pump so that they could be tube/bottle-fed when I was not there.*'

Olivia's first child was a delight to feed: '*So when I found I was pregnant with twins two years later I'd had a positive experience to convince me I definitely wanted to breastfeed again. However, I had a lot of opposition from var-*

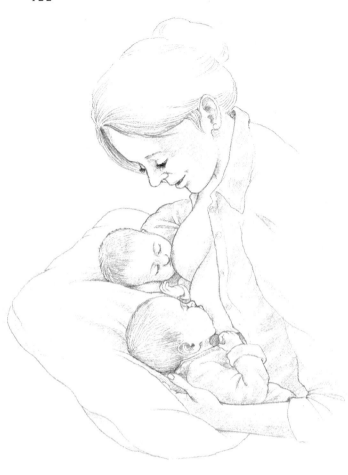

ious people fearing that Briony would somehow miss out, or I wouldn't have enough milk. The NCT came up trumps since I was lucky enough to have a breastfeeding counsellor in my area who had herself breastfed twins.'

Often a mother has to contend with the serious doubts of 'the experts': *'All the medical staff were very sceptical about breastfeeding twins. Thankfully I was in contact with other mums of twins who had succeeded and enjoyed it, so I was absolutely determined to go ahead. I read everything positive about feeding twins and ignored all else. I had to keep reiterating to my consultant that I was not going to try breastfeeding both, but that I was going to.'*

AN ADDED complication for you as the mother of twins may be that your babies are born early: prematurity is common with twin births. This factor may complicate the establishing of breastfeeding. If the babies are too small to suckle, you will need to express your milk until they can go to the breast. It is important that your carers understand your desire to breastfeed and give positive help and encouragement from the start. Sometimes, if the babies are near to term, the birth may be so tiring that thoughts of putting babies to the breast are far from being uppermost in your mind.

It certainly was for Simone: *'The birth of our babies was a very exciting and wonderful event, if rather shocking as the doctor produced a fourth baby on delivery. My first words on receiving a fourth healthy baby are not repeatable, and only made acceptable due to the colourful language of the three <u>not</u> four paediatricians present at the birth.*

I began to express breast milk about 30 hours post-delivery, which was the earliest I could possibly have tried to do anything apart from sleep and burst into tears.'

Helpful and supportive carers are essential in the early days, says Pat: 'It wasn't until I had been transferred to a room as a postnatal mother that I endeavoured to give the twins their first feed. The night-shift nurses had just come on and I was fortunate to be assigned a particularly helpful and support-ive nurse. She hunted out some cushions and a V-shaped pillow which I placed across my lap, supporting the babies, allowing me to feed them both at once.'

IN COMMON with other mothers, mothers of twins need good sup-port and positive encouragement in the early weeks of breastfeeding. You will also need good practical help during the learning phase. Positioning two babies together may seem an insuperable hurdle to begin with.

Establishing breastfeeding with twins (or more) may at times seem an impossible task, not always made easy by those around you, as Hilary remembers vividly: 'I insisted on being helped to feed each twin immedi-ately after birth and again later. I knew from my long spell on the antenatal ward that although breastfeeding was officially encouraged, staff were very apa-thetic and ready-made bottles were proffered at every opportunity. They assured me I'd have to supplement with bottles. I asked them to just let me get on with it. I started feeding one baby at a time, keeping one breast for each so that my supply would adjust to their individual needs. I kept one twin on each side of the bed. When he was there, my partner would walk up and down jig-gling one baby while I'd feed the other, then swap, but the waiting baby would scream constantly and this was hell. Many a nurse appearing at the door with a bottle of formula would get short shrift.

When my partner had not been there for a few hours and I was at my low-est ebb, they insisted on feeding soya milk through a nasal tube as I would not let them give a bottle. The babies were sick and pulled the tubes out, so I decided to try feeding them both at the same time. A friend with twins had lent me a V-shaped pillow to put across my front to rest them on – this was the single most useful thing and made keeping both babies in the right place much easier (recommended for all breastfeeding twins). Until I and they got the hang of it, keeping both latched on was very hard, but the peace when we did was bliss and the sensation of simultaneous feeding was wonderful – no dripping breasts, and less slow as well.

Thereafter I stuck to this in the daytime, calling a nurse to hold one while I got the second latched on – by this time the staff had realised I was going to manage somehow and were more helpful and quite impressed.'

At first Pat found it rather difficult to relax: *'Both babies seemed to be balanced on the pillow and I had only one pair of hands but two newborns. I found the night times difficult during these first few days. I seemed to be up and down all night long feeding one or other of the twins. Unfortunately, one or two of the nurses were unsupportive, critical even. One nurse, herself the mother of twins, repeatedly told me to "get them on the bottle". I felt very*

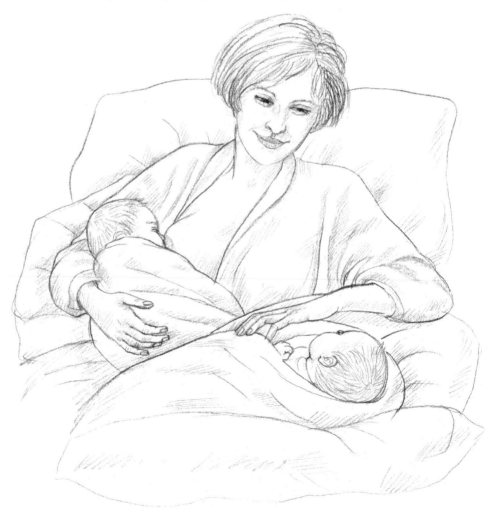

upset and isolated, indeed all the other girls in the adjacent rooms had single-tons and all these babies were bottle-fed. I felt as if I was just being awkward or bloodyminded.'

ONCE YOUR babies are home, adapting to your new additions can take a little time. Mothers of twins quickly learn to accept all offers of help and discover their own ways of coping with maintaining the daily routine. Feeding the babies together or separately, picking up and holding two small babies, coping with a lively toddler as well, are all common hurdles for a mother of twins to contend with.

Pat spent seven days in hospital and within that time her milk supply was established and was bountiful. Her twins had settled into a four-hourly regime – and they were both synchronised into the same regime: *'I never did get the hang of feeding two at once. One of the twins always fed a little less and always brought up a few mouthfuls afterwards. Once home I evolved a procedure for feeding whereby whoever awoke first was offered my fullest breast. In the meantime, the other baby was placed in a lit-tle rocker which I gently moved with my foot. When the first baby was fin-ished feeding, he swapped places with his twin and the second baby got my second breast.'*

Once Olivia's twins were home she experimented with different positions but decided to feed her babies one at a time: *'The main dif-ficulty I found when feeding them simultaneously was that I had a tremendous drop in blood sugar and my speech would slur and I felt faint. I had to sit with milk and a sandwich for me! I did feel very proud that I was able to satisfy two babies! However, it was clear that Ruth and Louise had different appetites. It was difficult to wind one baby whilst feeding the other. Also, I had decided to give the babies one breast each (Louise on the left and Ruth on the right!) which meant that Ruth had the most "difficult" nipple. When I'd tried to swap them around, I became hopelessly muddled and I was worried about one baby getting too much / too little hindmilk. So I began feeding them indi-vidually. I felt it was a special way to communicate with each individual.'*

Meg discovered that it was easier for her to feed both twins together: *'I was finally allowed to bring the twins home at six days old, having spent five weeks in hospital before and after the birth. The days and weeks all ran into one long blur. I was breastfeeding on demand which fortunately was going fairly well after a few false starts. I had eventually come to the conclusion of one baby always feeding from the right side and the other always on the left. With different demands I could sometimes be a bit lop-sided but each baby established its own supply. I found it easier to try and mostly feed them at the same time where possible because they were feeding almost hourly at first because of their size and then every two hours, otherwise I would be feeding 24 hours a day. The knack of getting them both latched on was quickly acquired, the art of sorting them out when one slips off and starts going crazy with milk spurting everywhere and still trying to hold and feed the other baby was not so simple. I found that Sophie screamed loudest, so it just became easier when this happened to take Jude off, restart Sophie and then let Jude resume his feed. Highly unfair, but it worked.'*

TIREDNESS SEEMS to be a constant factor for a mother of twins, especially if there is already a child in the family, as Meg found: *'There were days, particularly in the first six weeks, when Jo was at work, going out at 8.30am and coming home around 10pm, when I did not know which way to turn. I remember one evening when both babies were screaming, having fed all day, Simon was crying on his bed and I sat on the floor with the babies in my arms and burst into tears myself. It was sheer exhaustion that had caused it. Most nights I would be woken up to eight times. They never woke at the same time at night.'*

NIGHT FEEDS may be busier than daytimes. Even when the babies want to sleep, your milk supply may not allow you the luxury of an uninterrupted night's sleep.

Pat found she had to continue to breastfeed at night: *'Even when the twins showed all the signs of wanting to drop night feeds I had to keep one of the twins – the hungrier twin – on a night feed. It was physically painful for me to go from dusk to dawn without feeding; my milk supply was good and feeding two babies during the day meant that I would quickly become over-engorged during the night.'*

It may come as a surprise to find just how much you need to eat in order to keep up with your body's needs. Making milk for two (or more) growing babies can consume a vast amount of calories.

Introducing solids, or gradually switching to formula feeding, or a combination of both, at around four months, helps some mothers like Pat: *'The twins started to take solids at four months, mainly because I was beginning to find it difficult to keep pace with the amount of food I had to consume. I seemed to always be eating. The day I ate a whole family-sized chicken for lunch and followed it with a dessert, then cheese and biscuits and only vaguely felt satisfied, I decided that perhaps I should introduce the twins to a little of solids.'*

Baby rice allowed Hilary to sleep a little longer: *'By nearly four months we were so tired and my partner and family were begging me to supplement with milk feeds as well, although I was expressing in the morning to give them in the late evening when I was most tired, but the babies were thriving and I really felt bad about "giving up". Much to my relief a different health visitor came, who was very reassuring, and she suggested a little baby rice in the evening would be better than resorting to bottles.*

Thereafter, after rice at about 7pm, they would sleep until the late night feed and then went through until 5 or 6am, when we took them into bed and let them help themselves, swapping babies in between, which was all done in a semi-doze. This extra sleep was all we needed and I really began to enjoy the whole experience.'

The pressure on mothers of twins to wean their babies early can be strong. Many people find it difficult to believe that you can provide all the nourishment for two babies' needs for any length of time. Olivia resisted the pressure as long as she felt she could: *'At eight months, worries about their weight and comments such as "Are you sure you have got enough milk to give them?" finally made me decide to swap to bottles. I do not regret the struggles since I felt that ultimately each baby had intimate, almost spiritual, closeness with me, whereas bottle-feeding would have meant that anyone could have fed them.'*

Those who have experienced the 'ups and downs' of breastfeeding twins are, like Hilary, persuasive in their arguments for its benefits: *'I am glad I persevered and still miss it now. Even at the dreadful four-month stage, when we felt there would never be sleep again, I never wished I wasn't breastfeeding. Once they were going a few hours at night it was a truly wonderful experience.'*

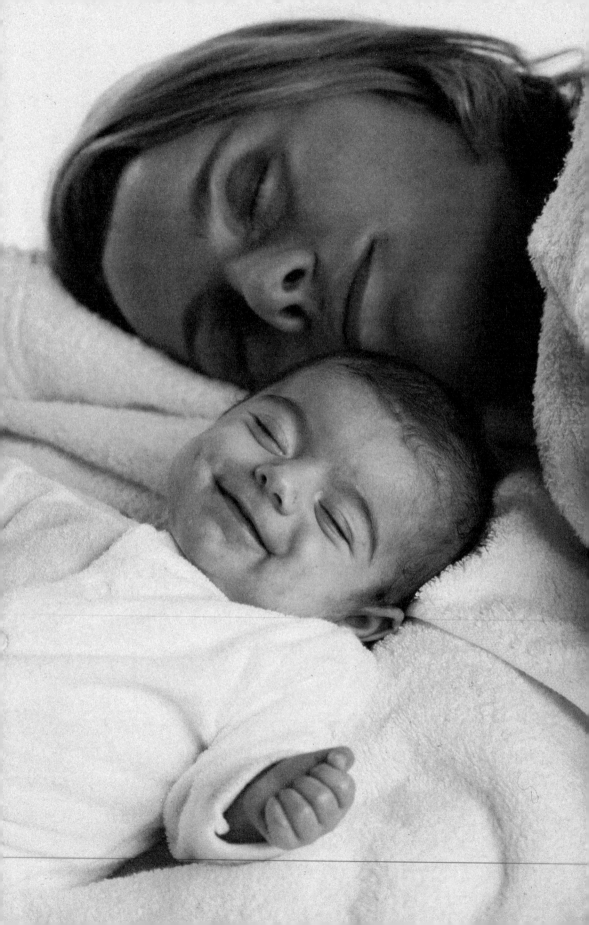

CHAPTER *eight* $Breast$
$troubles$

YOU MAY very well find that breastfeeding is 'plain sailing'. Problems are by no means inevitable. However, some mothers discover that there are minor irritations to cope with, or major setbacks which seem to spell the end of breastfeeding. Almost all the problems which arise during breastfeeding have solutions. In many cases, self-help methods are as important as medical interventions. Sometimes self-help is more important to you as you become more aware of how your breasts react – you can often act to prevent things deteriorating too far.

As with every other aspect of child-rearing, there are plenty of people with solutions to offer. Often, it is hard to decide which suggestions are best, and the same ideas do not seem to work for all mothers. This is probably because each breastfeeding pair is unique. No one breastfeeds quite like you and your baby do, so your ways are likely to be different to those of other breastfeeding pairs. This does not mean that your remedies are better or worse than anyone else's – if they work for you, that's fine. If you follow your own instincts, and maybe the suggestions offered earlier in this book for dealing with conflicting advice, you will find what works best for you and your baby.

PAINFUL NIPPLES

THERE ARE plenty of horror stories around about women suffering immensely in order to breastfeed. Some women will hear these tales of woe before they themselves begin breastfeeding, as Laura did: *'My own mother breastfed me for six weeks and had always said that it hurts like knives the whole time. I had thought that that might happen to me and that I wouldn't put up with that kind of pain.'*

FEEDING FILE

Sore and cracked nipples: some suggestions

● Ask someone you trust to check your baby's position at the breast, especially if your baby is very young

● Change the position in which you feed your baby – try feeding lying down or with her tucked under your arm

● Try expressing some milk before putting your baby to the breast. Stimulate your let down reflex so your baby has less work to do at the beginning of a feed

● Express a little milk after your baby has finished feeding, and gently rub it round your nipples and let it dry

● If you are using creams or ointment, try stopping using them – they may be making the soreness worse

● Try feeding from the less sore side first

● Avoid using soap on your nipples – it is very drying

● Remember to release the suction first if you need to take your baby off the breast

● If you have been offered a nipple shield, try to use it as little as possible. Your baby will not be able to take as good a 'mouthful' of your breast with the shield, and this may increase your soreness rather than decreasing it. The shield also reduces the flow of milk, so long-term use will lead to a reduction in your supply

● If your nipples appear to be white and 'blanched' when your baby comes off the breast, this may be caused by poor circulation. Some women suffer from Reynaud's syndrome, which may also cause this blanching. Try drinking tea and keeping your breasts warm.

IN THE first seven to ten days some women do experience nipple sensitivity and/or painful breasts. A baby breastfeeding effectively and feeding whenever he wants usually results in this discomfort being short-lived. Unfortunately, for some women like Susy and Leah this condition does continue into the following weeks.

'For the first two and a half weeks I suffered badly from cracked nipples. This problem meant that I never enjoyed feeding and would put off the dreaded moment until my baby was absolutely starving! I think it was a self-perpetuating problem, in that when my baby was hungry she sucked all the harder. Also, probably my milk flowed less because I felt so tense.'

'One suggestion I read was to feed from the least sore side first as the baby would suck harder when she was hungry. I found that feeding from the most

sore side first worked better, as Ruth was inclined to play about with the nipple towards the end of a feed. Also, with the worst agony over at the beginning I found it easier to relax and enjoy the rest of the feed.'

WITHOUT SUPPORT, correct information about positioning and understanding, you may find it really difficult to find a feeding position that does not traumatise your breasts. Many try all sorts of remedies in desperation to find some relief for their pain. Elaine experimented: *'I tried most things – hot flannels, going topless, expressing with a pump (agony). Rotersept spray (no help and painful on my cracked nipples), Kamillosan ointment and rubbing my breast milk on my nipples. I also tried different positions and taking my baby off my breast until the latch looked OK but both my husband and I found it difficult to see his lower lip. The more I tried to experiment the more frustrated and angry he got.'*

Happily there is skilled, sensitive support available if you need it, as Hilary found out: *'The nipples both cracked and when I got home after five days, feeding became increasingly painful. There were sweats before a feed because I knew it was going to hurt so much; David would get upset, I would get upset. Matthew was such a great help to me at this time – he calmed us both down and encouraged me to contact the breastfeeding counsellor. I was so surprised that she was prepared to take time with us straight away. She watched how I fed David then helped with getting me more comfortable and David better positioned. We had several tries before there was any difference, but how much more relaxed I felt! There was someone who seemed to know what she was doing and gave the impression that she would sit there all night with me if necessary. It was so reassuring. Eventually we reached a position where David began to feed and it just didn't hurt – I really didn't believe it was possible until it happened. It was wonderful. A lot more chat from the counsellor, reassurance etc. and we went off home. It was more difficult at home, but with the newly-found confidence of knowing that it was possible for it not to hurt, I was prepared to take David off and try again until it worked. It took about a week for the cracks to heal on both sides.'*

SOMETIMES, NIPPLE shields are offered to mothers with sore nipples. The shields may alleviate the pain and allow the crack to heal, but they will not tackle the source of the problem and they may bring new difficulties. The breast cannot be milked as efficiently through a shield. Your baby will not be able to take as large a mouthful of breast as he can without it, so the baby receives less milk at each feed, and over time the mother's milk supply may be reduced.[51, 52] Some babies refuse to feed without the shield when it is removed.

Janice found nipple shields a mixed blessing: '*There was no obvious reason why my nipples had cracked. Michael's latch looked correct but felt wrong, perhaps his small mouth didn't open wide enough, perhaps I was holding him along the wrong arm. The midwife suggested I could use nipple shields until the nipples healed – it took four days. I was keen to resume direct breastfeeding and I was concerned lest Michael lose the technique of latching on to the breast. I started back on the breast a little at a time. Four days later, just as I was ceasing to use the shields, my nipples cracked again. I solved the problem when I altered completely the way I held Michael.*'

To Liza the shields seemed the perfect solution, until she discovered some of the hidden drawbacks: '*When my first baby was born my local hospital midwife fixed me up with a nipple shield to help my baby suckle in the first few days. However no one thought to warn me that my baby would become so used to the shield that he would reject the nipple. On top of this, it would seem that the nipple shield was cutting down the amount of milk my baby was getting.*'

Bethan found she needed the nipple shields and it took her a long time to manage without them: '*The nipple shield is a revelation, in more ways than one. Yes, I can now feed on the sore side with the shield, but I can also see now that the nipple is actually bleeding during a feed. I find the sight of bloody milk collecting in the shield while the baby comes up for air to be very disturbing. Feeding at home continues with reasonable success and relative comfort using the shield. The local midwife tried to convince me that 48 hours is long enough for the crack to heal, that the baby wouldn't feed well enough with the shield – so I tried without. The pain reduced me to such a state of tears and distress that the midwife almost fled in embarrassment. In fact it took the best part of two weeks before I was emotionally ready to try without the shield and three weeks to say that I was OK again. I am now just over seven weeks into motherhood and still breastfeeding. I am feeding on average eight times a day – and usually use the shield on either side at least once a day.*'

Thrush

Nipple soreness may develop due to reasons other than positioning, such as thrush or dermatitis. Help from a health professional or breastfeeding counsellor may be needed to identify the cause of the problem and to find an effective solution.

Pam's son Darren developed oral thrush: *'He had been prescribed anti-biotics at the hospital for an asymptomatic infection of the navel. The thrush wasn't bothering him at all, but obviously it needed treating. This involved drops four times a day for Darren and cream on my nipples twice daily. The thrush recurred, several times, and eventually after several courses of treatment, a hospital referral and a hefty dose of treatment for both of us, we got rid of it. Although I am prone to thrush, seven months into feeding my second baby it has not occurred at all.'*

It is important that, once thrush has been identified, both you and your baby are treated. Thrush likes warm moist conditions, and a mother's nipple in a baby's mouth provides the perfect medium for growth. Sometimes the treatment may take some time, as it did for Jane with her third baby: *'At six weeks my nipples became a bit sore – I looked in the baby's mouth to see white spots. Two prescriptions of Nystan drops failed to shift it, then I got Daktarin oral gel which worked practically overnight. I used Daktarin cream (prescribed for baby's bottom) on my nipples. A doctor friend suggested this, not my GP.'*

Jane also developed thrush when her fourth baby was very young: *'My nipples got worse instead of better. By day ten I was in tears at every feed, such was the pain. Thrush crossed my exhausted mind, but I dismissed this, stupidly thinking I/we could not have got it this early – where from, etc. A friend asked if I had looked in the baby's mouth – I hadn't. The baby's next awake period coincided with the first visit from the health visitor, so we looked and found lots of white spots. The baby had been difficult to latch on – no wonder! I looked at my nipples later – I couldn't believe I hadn't noticed the mess they were in. Bright pink fiery skin all over the nipples and radiating out over the areola – like star shapes. My health visitor phoned my GP from my house and oral gel was prescribed for Claire's mouth – nothing for me! I used the cream I had from a previous bout of thrush after feeds. I also used vinegar*

BACKGROUND NOTES

Thrush

Many people have candida albicans, the yeast responsible for thrush infection, on their skin without any problems. Most of the time it does no harm, but sometimes it can multiply and cause infections. Antibiotics kill bacteria, but they may also kill the bacteria which keep these infections at bay. They do not kill the yeast, so it is able to multiply freely. Thrush infections can develop more easily in people who are under stress, or eating a poor diet, are run down or anaemic. Thrush is easily passed from mother to baby, or from baby to mother.

Recognising thrush

● On the nipple – white spots on the nipple, red and sore nipples which do not clear up, itching and scaliness
● In the baby's mouth – white spots which do not rub off
● A sore red nappy rash can also indicate thrush
● Pain deep in the breast, throbbing in the breast between feeds, and pain during feeds, may be indicative of thrush in the milk ducts.

Suggestions which may help

● Thrush likes alkaline conditions, so soap should be avoided – use neutral cleansers instead, or just plain water
● A teaspoon of bicarbonate of soda in a cup of warm water makes a weak acid wash which will discourage the thrush
● A tablespoon of vinegar in a glass of water can also have the same effect
● Natural, live yoghurt contains bacteria which act against thrush – it can be smoothed on to the nipple, which is soothing
● Keep the nipples dry, as thrush likes moist, warm conditions
● Antifungal cream is now available over the counter from pharmacists. Ask for a cream suitable for nipple treatment.

When to seek medical help

● As soon as the condition is suspected – thrush is unlikely to clear up without medical treatment.

Likely medical intervention

● Antifungal cream, gel or drops
● It is very important that both mother and baby are treated together, even if only one is showing symptoms, due to the high probability of cross-infection
● Thrush in the duct may be treated with antifungals applied to the nipple
● Some people have found that a course of antifungal Nystatin taken orally works for thrush in the ducts
● Thrush is very persistent, and treatment lasting several weeks may be necessary.

Avoiding recurrence

● In cases of recurrent thrush, it is worth checking other areas which are common sites of infection, such as the vagina or the baby's bottom. Treatment for the whole family may be necessary
● Avoid antibiotics if possible; if they are needed, antifungals should be used at the same time.

solution at odd times and gave my nipples a lot of fresh air. I used nipple shields, but they barely took the edge off the pain. The thrush cleared up after about a week – it was wonderful to be enjoying feeding at last! It did recur a few weeks later but I noticed quickly and still had the cream and gel ready to use.'

Other causes of soreness

OCCASIONALLY, SORENESS may be caused by other skin conditions, such as dermatitis or eczema. These can be more difficult to treat, as Jennifer discovered: *'We did get off to a difficult start with sore nipples which progressed to sore areola, and after treatment for suspected thrush it was decided I had eczema. I then found myself using hydrocortisone cream which, of course, had to be washed off before each feed. By the time my baby was seven months old, my skin was improving and I gradually managed to do without the hydrocortisone.'*

SOMETIMES, YOU may find that your nipples become sore again, once the early days of feeding are over. There could be several reasons for this. Your baby may be teething and her saliva may be temporarily more acid; you may be pregnant; you may be about to resume menstruation. Whatever the cause, it is nearly always a very temporary condition. Jennifer describes her symptoms and the surprise she got when she discovered the cause: *'When Carol was about nine months old, I started to find feeding her really painful again, very much as it was in the early days. It was enough for me to be swearing or nearly in tears when she wanted a feed. I wondered whether it might be a sign of pregnancy and actually tried a home pregnancy test. A few days later, I had the start of my first period since she had been conceived.'*

PAINFUL BREASTS

Blocked ducts and mastitis

SOMETIMES ONE or more of the milk ducts becomes blocked. This may happen suddenly, after several weeks of trouble-free breastfeeding. A lump can be felt, which may be tender. These lumps are caused simply by obstruction of the duct, which prevents the milk

Use gravity to help the milk to flow.

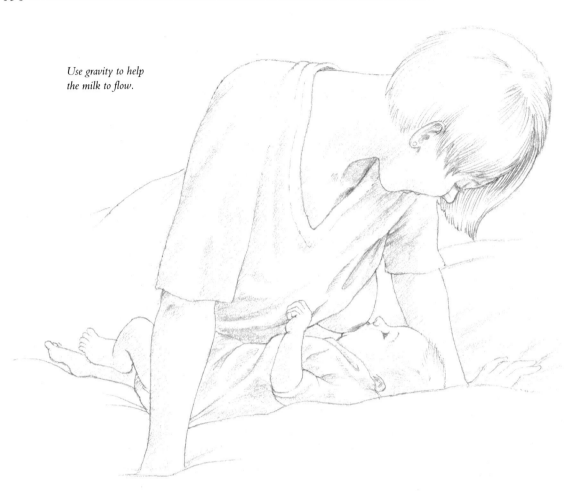

from flowing through. Common causes are too-tight bras; sleeping in a bra – if there is any movement of the bra it can press into the breast tissue – or even just your arm, if you sleep in an awkward position; or bruising from a cuddle from an enthusiastic toddler. Blocked ducts need prompt treatment, if they are not to develop into mastitis, but fortunately they do respond well to self-help.

Sheila found feeding her baby was the best cure: *'Just when I was getting the hang of things I started to get blocked ducts. This was very painful and for me, by far the worst thing about breastfeeding. I had lumps, very tender and sometimes covering a third of the breast for two to three days. I used a warm compress and painful massaging. I tried a breast pump with little success. Usually the lump would go suddenly while Helen was feeding.*

BACKGROUND NOTES

BLOCKED DUCTS

Recognising a blockage

● Lump you can see or feel
● Tender area
● Milk solids may be seen emerging from the nipple as a small white spot, or you may see a white blister on the nipple.

Suggestions which may help

● Feed the baby first from the 'lumpy' side
● Feed with the baby's chin nearest to the lump, so his lower jaw can strip the lump more effectively
● Use gravity to help the milk to flow – lay the baby on his back and hang the affected breast over him
● Massage the breast gently
● Warmth may help the milk to flow
● Using a wide-toothed comb lubricated with soap or baby oil, and firm but gentle pressure, stroke the breast over the lump towards the nipple
● Express milk after a feed if the breast still feels lumpy

● White spot or blister on nipple may need extra attention – a sterilised needle may be used to gently help it out if nothing else will shift it.

Has it worked?

● Lump should gradually reduce in size and tenderness
● May take a few days to disappear.

When to seek medical help

● If the lump does not respond to any of the above treatment within a few days.

Avoiding recurrence

● Check bra and clothing to make sure they are not too tight and putting pressure on the breast tissue
● Check baby's position at the breast
● Check that fingers are not pressing into breast tissue when feeding
● Change feeding positions regularly
● Avoid wearing a bra in bed.

Sometimes I would have a lump every week and it depressed me. This carried on for four months – I was very close to giving up. Just when most people seemed to be stopping feeding (about four months) I felt things were starting to go well and began to enjoy it.'

Sometimes self-help works well, as it did for Jean: *'I still had to be careful of blocked ducts if I used breast shells too often, or wore a smaller bra. But the second time this happened I prevented it getting worse by using the arm-swinging exercises, and "combing" my soaped breast, ideas the breastfeeding counsellor had given me.'*

BACKGROUND NOTES

Mastitis

Mastitis is inflammation, *not* necessarily infection. Milk from a blocked duct may have leaked into the breast tissue. The body thinks this is an infection and reacts in the same way, by increasing the blood supply, producing the inflammation and redness. Infection in the breast produces the same result; there is no way to tell if there is any infection present apart from analysing the milk to look for bacteria.

Recognising mastitis

● Red inflamed area on the breast (or whole breast)
● Breast feels sore
● You feel 'fluey' – aching, shivery, high temperature, tired and weepy.

Suggestions which may help

● Carry on with breastfeeding, even if advised to stop – this can make things worse
● Feed the baby more frequently, and use a breast pump if the baby is not taking all the milk available
● Feed from the side which is sore first
● Use the suggestions for treating a blocked duct
● Arm-swinging exercises will help to stimulate the circulation (scrubbing the floor or washing the windows will do as well)
● Rest if feeling unwell
● Alternate warmth and cold – warm flannels or warm water splashed on breasts, or a warm shower or bath, especially before a feed; cold compresses (a packet of frozen peas, or ice-cubes wrapped in a clean tea-towel are good) after a feed will help to reduce the inflammation.

Has it worked?

● Self-help techniques should work in 12–24 hours

● Fluey feelings should subside and inflammation reduce.

When to seek medical help

● If self-help techniques produce no improvement in 12–24 hours or earlier if you are worried
● If mastitis keeps recurring.

Likely medical intervention

● Antibiotics (check compatibility with breastfeeding – you do not have to stop breastfeeding whilst taking most antibiotics)
● Baby may develop irritability and/or diarrhoea, due to antibiotic passing into the milk – this is not dangerous, but the baby may demand more frequent feeds if she is thirsty
● Some mothers find that eating live yoghurt helps to avoid the thrush which can sometimes develop whilst they are taking antibiotics.

Avoiding recurrence

● Check positioning of the baby at the breast
● Change feeding position regularly
● Cutting down on saturated fats and avoiding caffeine (tea, coffee, cola etc.) may help
● Avoid sprays and creams applied to the nipples, which may affect the skin's natural barriers
● If mastitis recurs more than twice, ask GP to take a swab from the baby's nose and throat – the baby may have an infection which is reinfecting you.

YOU MAY find that you develop a blockage at the very end of your nipple, which looks like a white spot or blister. This may be an accumulation of milk solids which have built up in a blocked duct. They can be stubborn, and may need special treatment to remove them in addition to the usual self-help techniques.

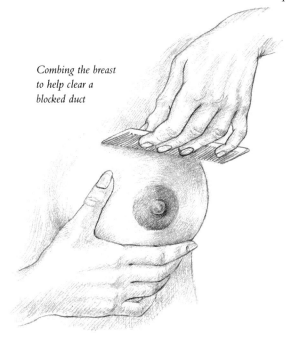

Combing the breast to help clear a blocked duct

Carol used knowledge acquired from training as a breastfeeding counsellor: *'I noticed a slightly tender area in my right breast, which felt as if it was just behind the areola. On examination, I discovered a tiny, white blister, probably no bigger than a pin-head, on the nipple. I could pierce the blister with a disinfected needle, but as I was experiencing severe pain by then, I didn't want to risk it, in case the pain became worse. Or it could be associated with a blocked duct and indeed, the area was becoming increasingly lumpy, though neither hot nor red, thank goodness. I therefore did everything I would normally do for a blocked duct and hoped it would get better soon! Sure enough, within three to four days it was better, but the blister had burst and dried up in the process.'*

BLOCKED DUCTS, left untreated, may develop into further breast inflammation, or mastitis. You may find that mastitis strikes very suddenly or it may develop gradually, often from a simple blockage. Mastitis simply means inflammation of the breast, and does not necessarily mean that there is an infection in the breast. If you go to your doctor with symptoms of mastitis, you will usually be given an antibiotic, as infection can develop rapidly, and the GP will be anxious to avoid an abscess developing. The most important part of treating mastitis is increasing the amount of milk flowing through the breast, preferably by feeding the baby more frequently. Interrupting breastfeeding at this time will only make matters worse.[34]

You may find that you can treat mastitis with the same self-help remedies which work for a blocked duct, but you may need a course

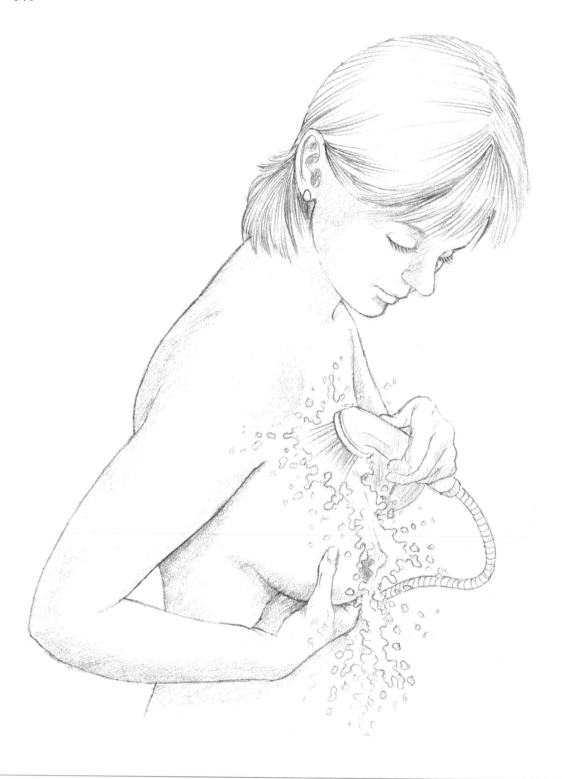

of antibiotics as well. Sometimes, though, taking antibiotics can have unwanted effects, on your baby as well as on you.

What is certain is that if you have mastitis, you will be feeling very low and miserable, like Julia: *'When Susan was five months old I developed mastitis. I felt fine all day, we had friends round in the evening and when they got up to leave I couldn't move! I tried all the self-help remedies I could and continued to feed. The doctor came out to see me the following morning and was very understanding. He suggested that I continue with the self-help but also prescribed antibiotics to be used only if I really needed them, due to the fact that they would be passed through in the milk. By that evening I felt so miserable that I started on the course of antibiotics. Within 24 hours Susan was miserable, had diarrhoea and a bad nappy rash. I stopped the antibiotics immediately and the mastitis soon cleared up, but Susan's nappy rash got so bad that it bled at nappy changes.*

I took her to the doctor's, who diagnosed thrush and prescribed cream to apply at nappy changes. Over the next four months the thrush continued and we had to make three repeat visits to the doctor for different creams. Had I realised the extent of the damage that the antibiotics could cause I most definitely would have avoided them.'

YOU MAY only have one bout of mastitis while you are breastfeeding, but some mothers seem to be prone to attacks. If this is the case, it is worth investigating a possible cause, such as an infection in the baby's nose, which can reinfect you if it is not noticed.

Many mothers become adept at spotting the first signs of mastitis, and manage to avert the attack without needing to take antibiotics, like Jackie: *'Whilst feeding Molly I had mastitis – twice, at nine and thirteen weeks, due I think to a small bra combined with a sudden unexpected increase in milk supply. After the second attack of mastitis I spoke to a counsellor who suggested altering feeding positions to help drain all parts of the breast, and to express milk if I was very full. A hand pump proved useless but I became adept at expressing by hand, leaning over a sterilised ice cube tray – letting the let down do all the work! By now I was always vigilant for lumps and this led to some very strange feeding positions (not possible in public!) and if I felt full I would quite often leave off my bra. I continued feeding Molly happily until she was nine months old, when she weaned herself.'*

Sore breasts

OCCASIONALLY, YOU may feel that your whole breast is sore and painful, but you do not seem to have the symptoms of mastitis. These pains may be due to thrush in the milk ducts, which can cause pain deep in the breast, but sometimes it seems that there is no obvious cause. It may sometimes be that you have not recognised mastitis, and you are diagnosed only after struggling on in pain for some time. This can happen if you have suffered sore nipples – it is not difficult to mistake the mastitis for a continuation and extension of your soreness, as Amy did: *'I developed cracked nipples on both breasts and feeding times became torturous. I had deep pains seeming to originate in my armpits which spread throughout my whole breast. This lasted throughout the whole feed. I often cried during the feeds as it was so painful – or before, in anticipation of the pain. I tried most things – hot flannels, going topless, expressing with a pump, Rotersept spray. I also tried different positions and taking my baby off my breast until the latch looked OK. The turning point came when I went home to my parents for Christmas when my baby was about three weeks old and my mother insisted I saw a doctor because my breast was inflamed. I was diagnosed as having mastitis and prescribed antibiotics. Within a few days the deep pain within my breasts eased and latching on became a great deal easier. By six weeks I had pain just on latching and by eight weeks I had pain-free feeding: two years and three months later I am still feeding Timothy.'*

Abscess

A BREAST ABSCESS is a very unpleasant condition, and any mother who finds that she has one may find herself needing several weeks to recover. Occasionally, an abscess responds to antibiotics without any further medical intervention, but more usually, the abscess is lanced and drained in hospital. Sometimes it may be aspirated. Jayne's experience is typical: *'After about seven weeks I developed a breast abscess. Before I knew this, I battled on through ever-increasing discomfort, believing it was just a blocked duct. Finally when I was driven to the doctor, mastitis was diagnosed, but after three sessions of antibiotics and a lot of pain I was in hospital. So large was the abscess that it needed a drain after the operation and two weeks of daily visits to hospital and then three times a week to the surgery*

BACKGROUND NOTES

Abstract

Abscess

An abscess may follow on from poorly treated blocked ducts or mastitis, especially if you have followed advice to stop breastfeeding. An abscess can also develop in the absence of any other symptoms.

Recognising an abscess

● Soft lump may be felt on breast
● Pus may be seen in the milk
● Lump may be painful, but may not
● You may feel ill, as with mastitis.

Suggestions which may help

● Breastfeeding can continue if the baby is not sick due to blood or pus in the milk
● Express milk from affected side and continue to feed from other side to maintain supply, if baby will not tolerate pus.

When to seek medical help

● Immediately – abscess is a medical condition which needs immediate treatment.

Likely medical intervention

● Antibiotics
● Lancing of abscess and draining or
● Aspirating of abscess – inserting a syringe and drawing off the pus – this may be done once or twice
● Aspiration is less traumatic and can mean less disruption to breastfeeding.

Avoiding recurrence

● If abscess has developed from untreated blocked ducts or mastitis, follow suggestions above for these conditions
● Avoid sudden weaning.

---

nurse before I was down to a simple dressing. Through all the weeks, I craved a shower or bath without bothering about spurting milk everywhere or getting dressings wet.'

BLOOD IN THE MILK OR COLOSTRUM

RARELY, DURING pregnancy, you may notice streaks of blood in the colostrum which leaks from your breasts. If there is a lot of blood, the colostrum may look like cold tea or coffee. For some women, this may continue after the birth without any nipple soreness or cracks developing.

Nadine was 16 weeks pregnant when her breasts started to leak: *'Shortly after this I was horrified to discover what appeared to be blood in the colostrum. I was especially concerned because to begin with only one breast was affected and I imagined all sorts of dreadful things. When the second breast also started to "bleed" I was actually quite relieved, it seemed to be more likely to be pregnancy related than cancer related, if they were both doing it!'*

This can be quite alarming, particularly as there does not seem to be much information about this in the breastfeeding literature. It may be viewed with some suspicion by health professionals, which could make you think that it is something sinister, as Lilian discovered: *'Two days after the birth of my first child I noticed, much to my horror, blood in the colostrum from my left breast. I mentioned this to the staff nurse straight away but no one seemed to have come across this problem before and consequently I received very little reassurance. In fact, this negative reaction made me feel even more frightened and I was convinced there was something seriously wrong with me.'*

Sandy also found very little reassurance from anyone: *'I was upset about the whole business, especially after talking to one of the local midwives, who said that blood in the milk usually made breastfeeding impossible as the baby would be sick all the time. During labour one or two of the midwives were startled to see "blood" on my hospital gown long before my son made an appearance. One went away and consulted her textbooks and came back to tell me that it was classed as a red-coloured discharge and not blood. Another said that she had seen it only once before in her career.'*

Most women find that the blood disappears as soon as the milk comes in and they continue to establish breastfeeding normally. Your baby will not be adversely affected by receiving the blood. Some women, like Liz, have found that they are advised to express and discard the milk from the affected breast: *'I saw the breast nurse on the ward and she was helpful, suggesting that I use the electric breast pump on the affected side until the milk was clear of the blood, but to continue feeding normally from the right breast. Once my milk came in properly the blood gradually disappeared until a final examination of my milk sample revealed I could now feed from both sides. What a relief!'*

Agnes found she was reassuring the nurses, rather than the other way round: *'After my son was born he was immediately put to my breast and we succeeded in breastfeeding quite quickly. He didn't have any problems with the taste as far as I could see, and he was not a "sicky" baby at all. It was necessary to reassure the nurses a couple of times, because on the odd occasion that he did bring milk back up after a feed during the first few days it was actually an orangey-brown colour! Fortunately, when the milk came in, it was normal and the "bleeding" stopped.'*

IT IS POSSIBLE that blood in your milk or colostrum is similar to a nosebleed. The cells lining the milk ducts are served by fragile capillaries (tiny blood vessels). Some of these may burst spontaneously or be caused to do so from over-enthusiastic expressing of colostrum. Very occasionally, the blood does not 'clear up'. In these circumstances, it is wise to consult a doctor to check whether there is any cause for concern.

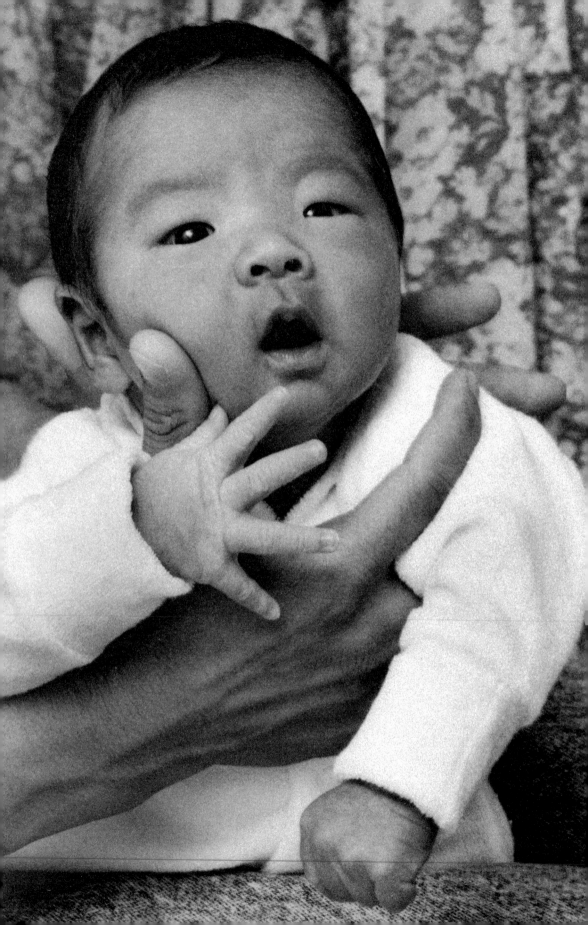

CHAPTER *nine* *Feeding difficulties*

SOMETIMES BREASTFEEDING itself seems to be going well, but your baby may become unsettled or difficult. You may wonder whether you are doing something wrong; you may worry that your breast milk is not 'satisfying' your baby – understandable concerns when you are solely responsible for your baby's nutrition. In many cases, there is no real answer, except perhaps that babies are people and have moods and emotions like adults, and are very good at expressing themselves, loudly. Sometimes, you will find a connection with breastfeeding and, once identified, the difficulty can usually be worked on successfully. Patience and experimentation are the keys to success.

CRYING BABIES

IN THE early weeks at home, you begin to understand and interpret your baby's 'language'. You try to establish how to respond to the cries of your baby. In responding to the baby's cries appropriately, you expect the crying to cease. It is a perfectly natural wish; it is distressing to listen to a baby crying. Perhaps we presume that, as the parents, we will be able to find the magic cure.

It seems as though there is some pressure on new parents to find the 'cure' as soon as possible. Well-meaning relatives might ask, 'Has the baby settled down yet?' This could mean, have you reached some understanding of your baby and can you respond to the baby so that there is not too much crying. There really is a desire for 'things to settle down' after the birth of a baby.

Generally speaking, 'things' do tend to get easier after the first couple of weeks, but, unfortunately, for some they do not. If you have to listen to the sound of your baby crying, knowing the repertoire of possible comforts does not result in peace for the baby and for you, it can be a trying time. Fortunately for most parents, the times of inconsolable crying are limited, but for some they do go on longer and bring considerable distress to all concerned. Mary's experience was distressing: *'All went well until she was about three weeks old and she began to scream all night long, feed on and off and would only stop crying when she was rocked. She would feed and settle for a short while and then begin screaming again. This was a difficult time for me and one when I wish I had been aware of the NCT and the existence of breastfeeding counsellors. However, I battled on determined that I was doing the right thing by breast-feeding although I was often given advice to the contrary. My mother-in-law told me that I should put her on the bottle as my milk was obviously too thin. I took Harriet regularly to the clinic and was assured by my sympathetic health visitor that she was fine and her weight gain was certainly enough, sometimes 1lb in a week. I badly needed this reassurance that there was nothing wrong with my milk supply or the baby and luckily this help was available. As time went on and Harriet still screamed most of the night, my health visitor suggested that I should limit feeding to about three-hourly intervals to prevent her from over stimulating my supply and giving herself tummy ache. I sought help from my GP but again only received reassurance that my baby was healthy but he didn't offer any particular advice or solutions. I resented the inference that my problems were a result of my incompetence and still felt that I was doing the right thing. Eventually, things did improve, she screamed less and fed less and slept more but the improvement was gradual. I did try to solve my own problems by reading as much as I could about feeding and crying babies but was never able to come to any conclusion about the cause of Harriet's crying. I did wonder whether she suffered any intolerance to dairy products she received via my milk but found it difficult to eliminate these foods from my diet and did not persevere for very long. I still do not know whether Harriet had colic or tummy ache or whether I had an overabundant milk supply.'*

MARY SEARCHED for an explanation which she didn't find. Fortunately she was able to continue breastfeeding, holding on to the belief that breastfeeding was the right thing for her and her baby. Not all women can be so confident about breastfeeding, particularly when faced with an unhappy baby as this seems to be very closely bound up with their own confidence and self-esteem.

The images of motherhood that many women have are often composed of fairly vague memories of their own mothers, mixed with the very powerful images from the media. Media images are pretty clear

FEEDING FILE

Ideas for comforting a crying baby

● Offer the breast, for comfort if not for food

● Tiny babies need to suck. Some babies need more sucking time than others. You may wish to provide an artificial comforter, such as a dummy. Be aware that sometimes these can affect a small baby's ability to suck at the breast

● She may suck a clean finger for a while

● Hold your baby near you. The heartbeat is a reassuring sound. Some babies like to be held upright, near your shoulder

● Many babies like movement – a rocking chair, or simple, natural rocking that men and women do when holding a baby

● Your baby may like gentle rhythmical patting or stroking. Caressing your baby may help him to feel secure

● Some babies like to be swaddled, an age-old practice. Lay the baby on a shawl, soft blanket or sheet and wrap him snugly, with each arm held down next to his body

● Warm water may be relaxing. Give him a bath alone or, even better, have a warm bath together

● Show him his reflection in a mirror. Babies are fascinated by faces. The mirror will give him a new angle on his mother or father

● The sound of his parents' voices gently reassuring him can be very effective

● Offer a different view or experience to your baby – a ride in the car or watching the washing machine go round, perhaps

● A continuous noise, like a vacuum cleaner, can soothe some fractious babies. Others may respond to womb-music tapes if these are introduced in the early weeks

● An older baby may enjoy kicking on a mat without his nappy

● An older baby may like sitting in a bouncy cradle-type chair and watching his parents

● She may enjoy lying in the pram in the garden – the leaves and clouds may be interesting to watch

● Sometimes your baby may cry because she wants to sleep, but is just too tired to be able to 'go off'. Holding her close, talking gently and staying calm may be enough to help her relax into sleep

● If you become overwhelmed by her crying, place her safely down in a cot or pram and leave her for a few minutes while you calm down

● Ask for some help, so you can have 'time off'

● Telephone a friend or a breastfeeding counsellor and talk about how you feel

● If it all seems to be getting out of control, contact a self-help support group, such as CRY-SIS. CRY-SIS Support Group, BM CRY-SIS, London WC1N 3XX. Tel: 0171 404 5011

● Ask your health visitor for support

● If you suspect that your baby may be sensitive to dairy products in your diet, ask a breastfeeding counsellor for the NCT *Cows' Milk-Free Diet Sheet for Breastfeeding Mothers.*

— happy, contented baby means a 'good' mother. A woman coping with a crying baby will very easily make the alternative link in her mind — unhappy, crying baby means a 'bad' mother. This can be utterly demoralising and you may come to believe that somehow the baby's crying is really your fault. A misguided comment, for example, that the baby is crying because of the 'nature' of your milk could leave you vulnerable to giving up breastfeeding altogether. Although in a strong moment you may know that it is not the case, it can feel like just too much 'blame' to carry.

COLIC

SOMETIMES PEOPLE may suggest that your baby's crying is caused by 'colic' or 'tummy ache'. There really is no consensus about what might cause the type of crying which is commonly described as 'screaming'. This crying does seem to be of a different 'quality' and sounds, to the parents, as though their baby is in distress.

Sometimes, an explanation itself can relieve you, even though you are still left having to cope with a crying baby, as Nina was: *'My son Josh, now nearly six months old, suffered from "colic" for the first twelve weeks of his life. Anyway, at first I enjoyed the closeness I felt when feeding Josh but as his colic got worse I found I felt guilty as if it was my fault that he was in so much pain and wondered whether there was something wrong with my milk. I went to the doctors with him, as I was, on a number of occasions, concerned that there might be something else wrong with him as he cried constantly day and night (well, not quite, but it certainly felt like it!). The doctor explained that she thought that as he was a big baby (he was 9lb 1oz when born) he would get very hungry and gulp his milk but get quickly full up with wind. I must also add that he never burped however much we tried to burp him and this was obviously part of the problem. He would start to feed and after just a few minutes he would start to cry and therefore couldn't take much milk. I began to feel desperate.*

Numerous people told me to "put him on the bottle" and that he was just hungry but I did not believe that this was the case (and still don't). I did find that I got very upset sometimes when feeding him as he was so unhappy and unsettled. My husband and I used to take it in turns to walk around the room carrying him — although it didn't seem to help Josh much, at least we felt we were doing something to try to comfort him. Anyway, I am glad to say that that all seems a long time ago now as he is a happy little soul now, but when we were told that this was sometimes called "three month colic", the three months certainly seemed a long time coming around!'

IF THE persistent crying occurs mostly in the evening, there have been suggestions made that it could be related to this being the busiest time of the day for you. Perhaps the baby is not receiving all that he requires in the way of food or comfort from you while you are occupied with other household chores. This might be particularly relevant for you if you have older children to care for. Some women consider this for themselves and adjust their way of life accordingly.

Paula did just that: *'Some evenings I found Charlotte very unsettled, crying, desperate to feed but refusing the breast. This, of course, is very typical behaviour in young babies. After some weeks I made a connection: I discovered that if I had skimped on my lunch or missed out a snack around tea time then Charlotte would yell the house down come evening.*

I expect most of us find late afternoon/early evening a busy time or even frantic time of day. I know I actually feel shattered by dinnertime! To overcome this low I took care to eat a decent-sized snack when I came home with Hannah from school. I prepared my evening meal earlier in the day or else bought easy ready-made dishes. I did any urgent tasks earlier in the day if I could, or just left them. This helped me to ease the pace at the end of the day.'

YOU MAY seek the opinion of the health professionals involved in your care. You may be concerned that there is something medically wrong with the baby.

Colette was able to link events retrospectively, after reading about possible food intolerances: *'At about ten days Graham developed severe infant colic. Like most first-time parents, we had never heard of this and were horrified to find there was apparently nothing we could do about it. We tried gripe water, Infacol, massage (not cranial massage, as there is no local practitioner up here) – all the usual ideas – to no avail. My health visitor could only suggest that I should avoid spicy foods, my breastfeeding counsellor offered her sympathies. My mother then told me of someone who had had a similar problem, and had found that it was caused by dairy products in her own diet. I gave up milk, cheese, and many other things – within a week the colic had gone. Each time I reintroduced even a tiny bit of milk, it returned – generally it would come on about 24 hours after I had eaten the offending substance, and take about three days to go, over which time Graham would scream in agony each evening, sometimes not stopping till 5am the next morning. In the end, I gave up all dairy products until Graham was weaned at eight months. I did not find this nearly so difficult as people seemed to think – in fact, cow's milk now tastes very odd! I did miss cheese in particular as our diet is normally mostly vegetarian, but this was a small price to pay for a colic-free baby, as anyone who has experienced it will agree.*

My main problem with the dairy-free diet was other people's attitudes; my health visitor just would not believe that milk, etc. was to blame for the colic, and kept on suggesting other possible causes – curry (her bête noire), orange juice, grapes. I also found that some health professionals, and NCT-ers, had known about the link between dairy produce and colic for some time, but had not suggested this to me as a possible cause. A Canadian friend recently passed on an article from a health visitors' journal citing research which has shown that at least one-third of babies with colic will show significant improvement if their mothers give up milk.[53] I feel that if people who knew about this had told me right at the beginning, I could have saved Graham several weeks of agony, and myself and my husband weeks of sleepless nights.

My breastfeeding counsellor did – after I isolated the cause of the colic – let me have a useful diet sheet which explained, in particular, the importance of maintaining a good intake of calcium on a dairy-free diet. For eight months I consumed quantities of sesame seeds and pilchards – not together! – to make sure that Graham's bones grew well and also that I didn't develop osteoporosis.'

THOSE BABIES born to families with a history of allergies are more likely to show sensitivity to various substances and cow's milk is one of the most likely allergens. Exposure to the allergen will result in some sort of reaction, commonly experienced as an unsettled, unhappy baby. It could be that your baby received a bottle of cow's milk formula in hospital, or an early top-up and this can be sufficient to sensitise the baby to the presence of cow's milk derivatives in your breast milk. In these circumstances, exclusion of all dairy products from your diet may bring considerable relief to you and your baby. If you think your baby may be reacting to something in your diet, it might help to talk to your health visitor or a dietician.

It may be that a crying baby is sensitive to something he is taking into his stomach either directly, for example, vitamin drops, or to something passed through your milk, for example, if you are taking vitamin drops or iron tablets. Faced with coping with a crying baby, many women review closely what the baby is receiving. Commonly, caffeine is cited as a possible stimulant and it is possible that if your overall intake of all caffeine-containing drinks exceeds five cups a day this could affect some babies adversely, making them more 'fussy' than usual. It does take about two weeks of exclusion of any substances from the diet to eliminate it reliably from your breast milk. You would need to persevere and exclude the substance from your diet to check out a suspected irritant to your baby. Again, check with your GP before starting any exclusion diet. It is sensible to discuss any exclusion diet with your GP, health visitor or dietician before starting. They may have useful suggestions for you. NCT breastfeeding counsellors may also be able to provide you with useful information.

If your baby's motions are consistently watery and green and she is not gaining weight well even though you seem to have plenty of milk for your baby, it could be that there is an imbalance between the foremilk and hindmilk the baby is receiving. The watery foremilk is rich in lactose and too much lactose stimulates the breastmilk to pass through the baby's gut too quickly.[54] She needs to receive both the foremilk and the fatty high-calorie hindmilk, so try if you can to allow her to finish the first breast first before offering the second. Later in the feeding relationship, she may prefer to take just one breast at each feed.

There may not be a satisfactory 'answer': some babies seem to cry despite every effort to calm them. Clearly the more support and encouragement you receive the better, until this phase of your baby's life passes.

BREAST REFUSAL

ONE OF the most distressing experiences which a breastfeeding mother can have must be when her baby refuses suddenly to feed from the breast, sometimes after months of happy feeding. It can seem as if the baby is rejecting her mother, not just the breastfeed, as Annabel recalls: *'My milk seemed to let down with great force, particularly on one side and Tracey would pull away choking and gasping for breath. She would often then refuse to feed again for some time as she was so upset. This made me feel a real failure. I wanted breastfeeding to be an enjoyable experience for both of us and instead I felt as if I was torturing my baby.'*

When Lee's baby, Simon, was nine months old, he had six teeth that he was so proud of – unfortunately he had taken to trying them out whilst feeding! One day he bit really hard and Lee reacted with an automatic "no": *'The following day Simon fed as usual but the day after he would not feed at all. He would burst into tears when I tried to latch him on and became very distressed. Initially I was unsure of the cause and thought through all the possibilities, such as change in the taste of the milk, smell, etc. Eventually I decided that it must have been my reaction when Simon bit me. Over the next few days we both became very upset. I felt so guilty that I might have put him off feeding completely. I expressed milk to give him from a cup as I wanted to maintain my supply. I had several comments from people trying to be helpful, such as: "He's nine months old, perhaps it's a good time to wean him." However well intended, these comments did not help as I didn't feel ready to wean him yet. Why do people always assume that mothers are looking for an excuse to stop feeding once the baby is six months old? I persevered and gave Simon a lot of love and cuddles and eventually on day five he began to feed again as if nothing had happened. Simon is now approaching his first birthday and is still feeding three times a day.'*

YOUR BABY may refuse to feed after a traumatic incident, such as Lee describes, or he may simply refuse to feed. He may kick and scream, fighting you as you try to offer him your breast. Each feed can become more difficult and the situation may last for several days. Usually, sudden refusal of the breast like this is not a sign that your baby is ready to be weaned from the breast. He is obviously distressed, but it may be difficult to pinpoint a cause.

Sometimes, your baby may be ill. Lee describes how her son reacted: *'When my second child was eight months old, he became ill and refused all food and fluids, including rejecting the breast. He became dehydrated and was in hospital. Most of the health professionals who I saw at that time did not understand why I was so upset at his refusal of the breast, but I felt that the most natural way to comfort my child was to breastfeed him and it was agony to see him screaming in pain and be unable to comfort him. Eventually the*

BACKGROUND NOTES

Breast refusal: possible causes

The reasons why your baby may suddenly refuse the breast may not be easy to uncover. However, there are some things which you can check:

● Positioning – check that your baby is correctly positioned at the breast

● Tongue-tied – if your baby's tongue is 'tied' to the roof of her mouth, she may find it difficult to breastfeed.

● Nipple confusion – if your baby has been given a bottle, this can confuse her. She may not remember how to suck at the breast, or she may find it easier to bottle-feed

● Nipple shields – sometimes suggested for mothers with sore nipples, these can lead to the baby becoming used to feeding through the shield and refusing the breast without it

● Thrush – a baby with thrush in his mouth will have a sore mouth and may find it painful to suckle

● Strong let down – if your let down reflex acts very rapidly and releases a sudden gush of milk, your baby may choke as he tries to cope with the fast flow. He may struggle and fight for breath and let go of the breast, coughing and spluttering. He may not want to repeat the experience

● Ear infection – if your baby has had a cold or snuffly nose recently, she may have developed an ear infection. This may cause pain when she tries to suck or swallow

● Sensitivity to something you have eaten – occasionally, your baby may react to something you have eaten or drunk, or to a medication you have taken

● Change in taste of breast milk – this may relate to the previous cause, as some foods, drink or drugs can alter the taste of your breast milk and your baby may dislike the new taste. Mastitis or a blocked duct may also alter the taste, sometimes only in the affected breast, and your milk may temporarily taste salty

● Change of smell – babies are very sensitive to smell. You may have changed your washing powder or fabric conditioner, or perhaps you have started using a new deodorant, shampoo or hairspray. Have you been given a new perfume recently? Your baby may be objecting to any of these

● Menstruation – your breast milk may alter slightly in taste or composition when you have a period. Some babies do not like to feed at this time, but return happily to breastfeeding once your period is over

● Teething – your baby's gums and jaw may be tender when a tooth is growing and he may be reluctant to feed

● A difficult age – once your baby reaches four to six months, he may be very easily distracted from the breast. He may also be very sensitive to noise around him and object to feeding in a noisy environment.

FEEDING FILE

Breast refusal: suggestions which may help

● Try to stay calm. Your baby is not rejecting you, and needs you to help him through this difficult time for him

● Talk to your baby; comfort her with a soothing voice

● Skin-to-skin contact is comforting. Try cuddling him close, but do not try to breastfeed unless he clearly wants to

● Try offering a feed when he is asleep or very sleepy

● Change the way you hold your baby: sit her up or lie down to feed

● Movement can be useful. Try rocking her, or walking around to feed. If you have a rocking chair, this may be soothing

● Try stimulating your let down reflex before you offer the breast. If your baby gets an 'instant reward' for latching on, she may continue to feed. This can be particularly useful if your baby has become accustomed to bottle-feeding, where she does not have to work for a let down. It may also help to remove the first 'rush' of milk if you have a strong let down reflex

● Express your milk to keep your supply going until your baby wants to feed again. You could feed the expressed milk from a cup until he is ready to go back to breastfeeding

● If you or your baby become distressed while you are trying to encourage her to breastfeed, stop and try again later. Fighting with her will only make the situation more tense

● If your baby has become 'addicted' to the nipple shield, try cutting the tip away, a little bit more each day, until you can feed without it

● Patience and gentle perseverance are the keys to success.

---

problem was diagnosed as a haemolytic streptococcus infection of the throat which was so bad he was unable to swallow. By this time he had not breast-fed for five days and although he received treatment which helped him very quickly, he now associated the breast with pain and screamed if I lifted my jumper as if to feed him. This was most distressing and I was determined to try to get him back on to the breast.

At first I just held him next to my breast when he was asleep, then gradually over several days I would put the nipple near his mouth and express a few drops on to his lips as he slept. Eventually one day he latched on in his sleep – I was ecstatic! Over the next few days I fed him when he slept, as he still went berserk if I tried when he was awake. Gradually he began to open his eyes while he was feeding. At first he pulled away and cried and I would com-

fort him, but one day he opened his eyes and kept feeding happily. This whole thing took about two weeks.'

BITING BABIES

WHEN YOUR baby's teeth begin to erupt, you may worry that your baby will bite you when he is breastfeeding. In fact, most babies get their teeth and continue to feed comfortably through this phase. Your baby needs to push his tongue out over his lower teeth when he is suckling. The 'danger' time is often when he has finished a feed and wants to 'play' at the breast. As he gets older, this playfulness may include a 'nip' at the nipple as he lets go the suction. Usually, a firm 'No!' is enough to deter him from repeating the game.

Patti's first baby bit her once: 'I said, "No!" loudly and firmly, and removed him. He never bit again. My second bit me several times, but usually after cutting a new tooth and she wore small 1–2mm square holes in my skin which were extremely painful. I persevered each time and once she readjusted her bite to accommodate the new tooth (three to six days) we were back to normal.'

You may find that there seems to be a connection between your baby biting you and something which affects you in another way, such as your periods starting or maybe something you are eating or drinking. This is usually a temporary problem, and may well solve itself, as it did for Debbie: *'When my daughter was exactly a year old, she started biting me at every feed (about three a day at the time). She would have her feed, then when she had finished she would get her teeth around my nipple and pull. She had never done it before and she stopped after a week.*

I then realised I'd just had my first period, and she had started biting me the day before the period started. She bit me again a couple of times when I had my next period and never did it again.'

RELACTATION

BREAST MILK is such a flexible resource that you can change your mind and begin to breastfeed again even if you have started giving bottles or have given up breastfeeding altogether. You can make this

---

FEEDING FILE

BITING BABIES

When your baby might bite

● Teething – teething babies like to chew on anything which may relieve their discomfort. Offering something cool to chew on before a feed may help. If you use a teething gel, make sure you don't numb your baby's tongue, which will make it difficult for her to latch on

● Slow let down – sometimes, your baby may want your milk to begin flowing more quickly than your let down allows. She may bite in frustration, to 'speed things up'. Check your positioning, as she will not be feeding efficiently if she is not well latched on. Try using warmth before a feed to help relax you and speed up your let down

● Attention seeking – your baby may want more of your attention than you are giving him when he is feeding, especially if he is older. Try giving him your complete attention; talk to him and look into his eyes

● Distraction/Lack of interest – if you try to feed your baby when she is not really interested, she may bite you if you are trying too hard to get her to latch on. If she is distracted when feeding, she may bite as she turns to look at whatever has caught her interest, holding on to the nipple with her teeth. You may need to feed in a quiet place for a while

● End of a feed – when your baby is coming towards the end of a feed, she may let go of the suction a little, and bite as she lets go of your nipple. You may be able to anticipate this by watching for her jaw tightening before she bites down. Try to release the suction gently so she has to let go properly

If your baby bites

● You will probably react strongly the first time your baby bites – you may scream or shout out and startle your baby. This may be enough to prevent recurrence

● He will not understand your distress and may be frightened by your sudden reaction, and may refuse to feed again. Try to stay calm

● Try not to pull her off the breast whilst she is biting down, as this will cause more damage. Slip your little finger into the corner of her mouth to try to release your nipple

● Say 'No' firmly and stop feeding

● If she persists, try putting her on the floor for a short time immediately after she bites. Most babies dislike being separated from you like this and realise that it is connected with biting

● If your nipples become sore, try the suggestions in Chapter Eight for soothing soreness

● Try and remember that your baby does not know she is hurting you and does not mean you any harm

● Show your baby how happy you are when she feeds and does not bite you

● Try pulling your baby very close to the breast, so that her airways are partially blocked and she releases your nipple to breathe through her mouth.

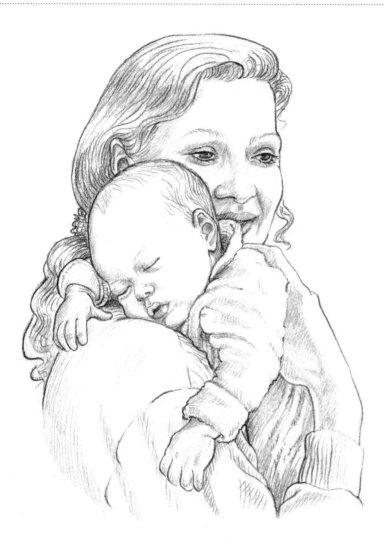

decision at any time after you have had a baby, although it will be easier if you start again within a few weeks of your baby's birth. It is even
possible to produce milk when you have not given birth, although in
this case, you may find it more difficult to stimulate a full supply for
your baby. Jenny managed to make the change from bottle to breast:
*'I couldn't breastfeed, it hurt, and part of me was convinced that if Simone
really was OK she'd have been able to suckle easily. Anyway, Simone fed bril-
liantly from a bottle. I knew she was sucking properly as I could see the milk
disappearing. I began to regret not breastfeeding her. Our first night at home
fuelled this as she screamed whilst my husband warmed her bottle – in hospital it had been in the room as I needed it.*

FEEDING FILE

Starting again – some suggestions

● Think positive: your milk supply can be built up again. It is even possible to make milk when you have not given birth, which some mothers do for their adopted babies

● Offer your baby a breastfeed before giving a bottle

● Use any of the suggestions in Chapter Four

for increasing your milk supply and cutting out complementary bottles

● A breast pump may be helpful to increase your supply – see Chapter Eleven for more suggestions about using a pump

● Contact your local breastfeeding counsellor for support and information.

Not really thinking there was anything I could do, I nevertheless rang a breastfeeding counsellor to ask her advice. She told me it was possible, and advised me to try feeding Simone at frequent intervals, but that initially I would need to top her up with formula until my milk supply got going again. By the time the midwife arrived that day, we were trying. Not without difficulty – Simone was enthusiastic enough but understandably confused, and I was having the same problems I'd had the first night in hospital although I was eventually getting her latched on.

It was difficult – Simone lost a lot of weight initially as after her first breast-feed she refused formula milk totally! I still had doubts sometimes that Simone was getting "enough" as I couldn't actively see milk disappearing from a bottle.

With help and support we got through the problems, and Simone was fully breastfed from then for 18 weeks, and continued feeding until she was eight months old.'

Jenny was able to breastfeed completely again within a short time, as her supply was still fairly good. If you want to start again after a longer interval, you may need extra help. A breast pump can be useful, to express milk and to give your breasts extra stimulation between feeds. There is also a useful device called a 'nursing supplementer', which Stephanie found to be very helpful: *'The breastfeeding counsellor brought round a feeding supplementer. The baby sucks formula from a small tube taped to the nipple, thus stimulating milk production. I started using it the next day. By the end of that week (Darren was now six*

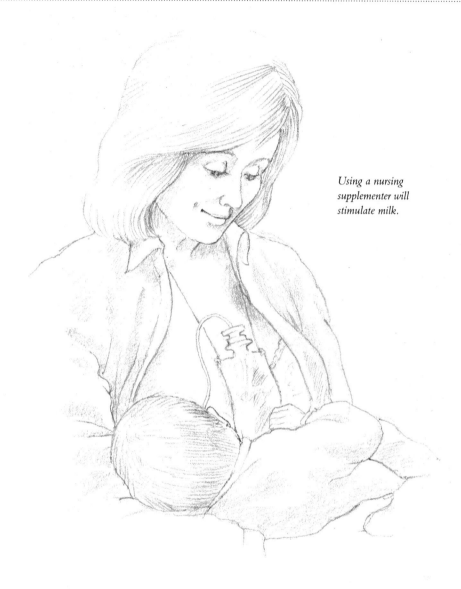

Using a nursing supplementer will stimulate milk.

weeks old) my breasts had enlarged noticeably and I could express small spurts of milk. It was enough to prove it was working. I felt so much better giving it a second try. Initially it had all become a vicious circle and bottle-feeding seemed a good solution under the circumstances. I feel great. It's only three days since he wouldn't do it at all, and now I can supply all his milk and he's so keen to take it. I'm so glad I made the effort to try again, but it wasn't easy, especially finding the right people to give advice. Darren is now a contented baby. We did it despite everything.'

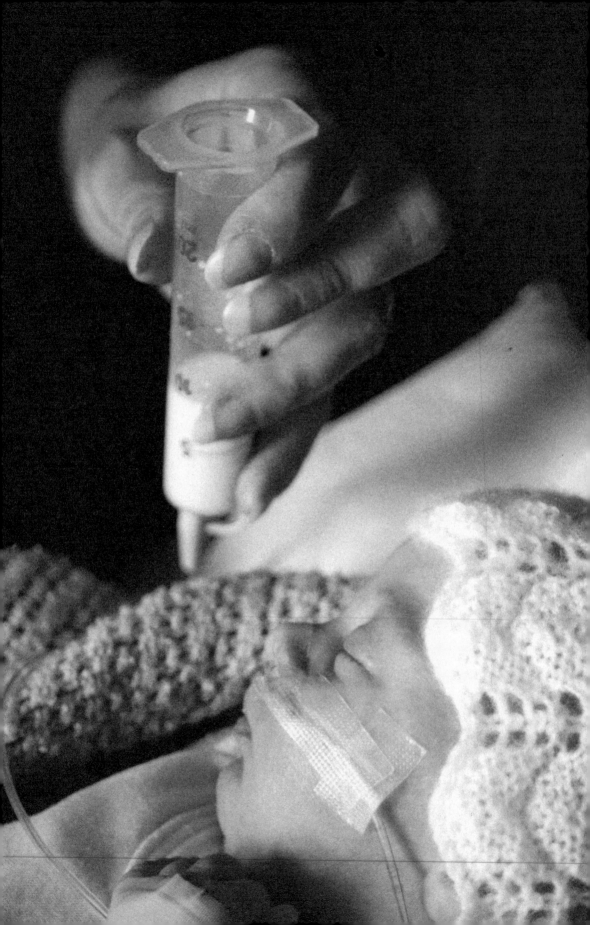

CHAPTER *__ten__* Breastfeeding in special circumstances

BABIES WITH SPECIAL NEEDS

SOME BABIES have special circumstances which have implications for breastfeeding. If your baby is premature, or ill, or has a disability, much effort may be needed to establish breastfeeding. Sometimes your baby may be temporarily unable to feed from the breast and you may need support whilst establishing and maintaining a supply of expressed milk which can be given to the baby by bottle, tube or cup.

Premature babies

IN 1990, 13% of babies were admitted to special care baby units (SCBU). The *Infant Feeding* survey[1] showed that mothers of low birth weight babies, that is babies less than 2,500g, are less likely to initiate breastfeeding. It seems that, even if you begin, the lower the baby's weight at birth, the more likely you are to stop breastfeeding. There are many reasons for this, not least the practical difficulties of your being on a postnatal ward and your baby being in the special care unit. For premature babies, breast milk is extremely valuable. Much research has been done on the benefits of breast milk for these tiny babies,[55] but this importance is sometimes not emphasised by hospital staff, who may be more anxious to put weight on the baby quickly.

Vanessa's son, Tony, was to stay in SCBU for five weeks and she used the pump virtually every three hours for much of that time: '*I was even more intent on breastfeeding Tony since I felt it was the only thing I could do for him. However, I produced very little milk and soon Tony's need for nutrition overtook my ability to supply – formula milk then had to be given; through a naso-gastric tube at first, then by bottle.*'

BACKGROUND NOTES

Milk for premature babies

Breast milk is important to premature babies. Studies have shown that giving premature babies their mother's breast milk reduces the chances of illness or death significantly.[56] The optimum growth and development of the brain is dependent on the baby receiving essential fatty acids through breast milk,[18] as is visual development.[20] The protective effect of breast milk is even more important in premature babies. Necrotising enterocolitis (NEC) is a rare but very serious disease seen in premature babies. It is very rare for a baby given breast milk to contract NEC.[23] Babies fed formula alone have a six to ten times higher risk of contracting this disease.[56]

However, establishing a milk supply when the baby may be too weak to suck at the breast is not easy. Some premature babies may be strong enough to suckle, but many will become exhausted if they attempt it. Others may not have developed a sucking reflex. In these circumstances, a fine naso-gastric tube is passed into the baby's stomach via the nose, and milk is fed to the baby via the tube. Breastfeeding itself is then introduced gradually, as the baby grows stronger and her muscle tone improves enough to suckle.

Kelly's first child was in special care at first for about four days, and it took tremendous determination to feed him: *'People kept saying: "Don't worry, it'll come — we'll tube-feed him for the present." But I knew it was most important (perhaps psychologically as much as physically) to put him to the breast whenever I could and he was remotely interested. He was sedated too — so people tended to make me feel it was silly to try, but my gut feeling was to put him near me, let him smell my breast, let him feel me near him, and give him the chance to root (and me to bond with him, I suppose). And suddenly one night, despite being sedated, he did begin to suck.'*

THE BIRTH of a premature baby is often a time of crisis; it is an extremely emotional time, and there may be concern for the baby's survival. You are not likely to be given the chance to feed your baby in the delivery room; you may hardly glimpse your baby before she is whisked away to special care. You are transferred to a post-natal ward, and may feel strange at being there without a baby, surrounded by new mothers with their babies. When you do see your baby in the incubator, she may be wired up to several machines. One of the best things you can do for your new baby at this time is to begin to express your milk.

Electric breast pumps are large, ugly and often housed in less than ideal places. Trying to get to grips with this weird machine, and to learn how to produce milk under such unnatural circumstances, is understandably difficult for all new mothers. A great deal of support and encouragement is needed, especially in the first few days when a lot of effort seems to produce very little in return. A thoughtless comment or passing remark can cause hurt and make some mothers want to give up the struggle, but a word of praise or encouragement will do wonders.

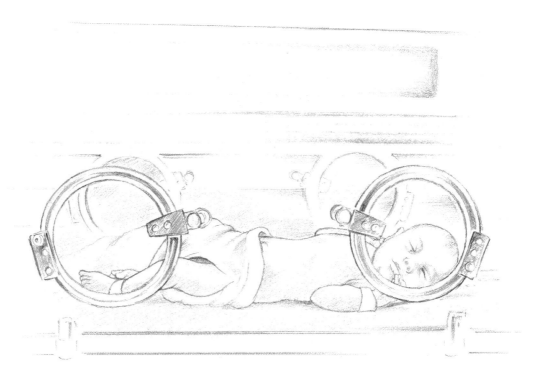

At 30 weeks' gestation Belinda had a second large blood loss and was whisked off to the labour ward: *'I was dilating quite quickly, unfortunately Karen was breech and I was told that a caesarean was safer for her as she was so premature. As I came round Nigel excitedly told me that we had a daughter in special care and first reports were good. It didn't take me long to fully come to and, after the usual clean up, was wheeled up to see Karen. She was 3lb 6oz and tiny – wired up and ventilated but she was ours and a healthy colour. The following day the midwife brought in a seemingly huge pump and we started the process of getting my milk supply going. I was determined to produce all that Karen required as, for the time being, this was all I could do.'*

Clare's son, Chris, was born five weeks preterm, before he acquired his sucking reflex: *'Throughout the day I kept asking about expressing and was constantly told there was plenty of time for that later. Chris was born at 9am and finally at about 9pm they agreed to get someone to show me how to use the breastpump. A male midwife showed me how to use the machine and how to wash out all the attachments, how to sterilise them, rinse them, and how to store and label the milk. During this unpleasant experience other*

FEEDING FILE

Initiating a supply of breast milk

● Initiating breastfeeding when the baby cannot suck at the breast is not easy but possible

● The most common method is to use an electric breast pump. Pumping needs to be started as soon as possible after birth, but you may not be in any condition to think clearly about this, so it is often 24–48 hours before anyone has time to suggest beginning to pump

● Most mothers do not let down well with the breast pump – it is hard, cold and mechanical, and gives you none of the stimulus that your warm, living baby does. A good prolactin response is essential for the body to start milk production, so this lack of prolactin response may be the reason for mothers producing a low volume of milk which is hard to sustain[57, 58]

● There are ways in which the response can be improved. Some experts have suggested that massaging the breasts before beginning to express[59] is one way of doing this. This will improve the supply of blood to the breasts, and stimulate the nipples – mimicking the skin-to-skin contact you have with your baby

● Stimulation will also induce a response from the other important breastfeeding hormone, oxytocin, which is responsible for the let down reflex

● An alternative to using a breast pump is to express milk by hand. This is commonly, and erroneously, thought to be difficult. Once the technique has been learned, hand expressing can be as efficient, if not more so, than using

a pump. There have also been suggestions that the fat content of hand-expressed breast milk is higher than that of pumped milk[58]

● Whichever method is used, it is important to start early and then to express regularly. The breasts need to have milk removed frequently in order to keep the demand/supply cycle going

● The rule of 'the more milk is removed, the more will be produced' holds true for expressing just as much as for breastfeeding. Many mothers do not express their milk frequently enough to keep the supply going: six to eight times in 24 hours is the minimum requirement, including one night-time session, when prolactin levels are at their highest[60]

● As premature babies only need a small quantity of milk at one time, it is useful to express the foremilk into one container, then express the remainder of the milk for the baby's immediate use. The foremilk can be used to 'top up' if necessary. In this way, the milk is likely to contain more fat, and therefore more calories, to help the premature baby to grow quickly. One expert suggests setting aside the first 25ml[59]

● Once the milk is expressed, it can be fed to the baby via the naso-gastric tube

● Some special care baby units are now also using special plastic cups to feed babies who cannot suckle at the breast from birth, but whose mothers wish to breastfeed when they can. The cup is used in preference to tube or

---

FEEDING FILE

bottle-feeding because it prevents babies from becoming confused between the different techniques of bottle- and breastfeeding

● The North Staffordshire Hospital introduced a new 'preterm infant feeding protocol' which was offered to mothers with newborn babies admitted to the unit who wished to breastfeed. This protocol involved massage, hand expression and frequent expressing, using tube or cup feeding until the babies were able to go to the breast. Using this protocol, the unit's breastfeeding success rate was raised from 1% to 58%[59]

● As soon as the premature baby shows any sign of being ready to suck, she should be encouraged to go to the breast

● Some hospitals prefer babies to progress from tube-feeding to bottle-feeding and then to the breast; others will allow the baby to go straight to the breast. It is commonly thought that bottle-feeding is in some way 'easier' than breastfeeding, but there is evidence that this is not the case.[61]

---

mothers were waltzing into the same room, taking disposable bottles of ready sterilised and made up formula; screwing on a disposable ready sterilised teat and walking out full of the joys of spring. Meanwhile I sat there, huge sore boobs attached to a hideous machine straight out of a physics lab. It hurt, it was embarrassing, and I produced no milk whatsoever, while my baby was in SCBU being fed formula through a naso-gastric tube by a nurse.

I desperately wanted someone to say: "Well done, you're doing the right thing for your baby, I know it hurts now but it will get easier, and you'll produce lots of milk and all will be well." I said it to myself instead.

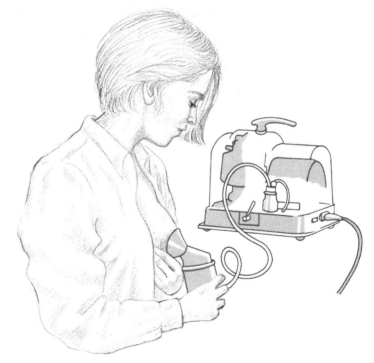

Three days of teeth-gritting pain and bleeding nipples later I produced one teaspoonful of colostrum and was elated. This was greeted by a passing midwife with, "That's no good, you'll need lots more than that."

In SCBU my contribution was treated more positively and was given to Chris as part of his next feed. I was delighted. They had more time in SCBU and kept helping me to put Chris to the breast before each tube feed. He couldn't really do it at all.'

TO BEGIN with, many premature babies are fed by a tube which is passed via the nose into the stomach – a naso-gastric tube. Once you are able to express your colostrum, then your breast milk, this can be fed to your baby via the tube. Very tiny babies do not need much food – a teaspoonful of colostrum can be a whole feed for a very small baby. Depending on the baby's condition, she may well be able to breastfeed at a later stage. As soon as the baby shows any desire to suck, you can encourage her to go to the breast. Even if she does not feed for very long, or very effectively, the close skin contact with your breast will stimulate your milk supply. Some mothers feel that the baby does not 'belong' to them; the baby is surrounded by machines and tended by special care staff. You may feel that you need to 'ask permission' to put your baby to the breast.

Suzanne was taught by her midwife to tube-feed the twins next to her breast, then gradually allow sucking at the same time, until their reflex was strong enough to remove the tube: *'Then I began trying to feed them both at once. I stayed in day and night for a few days to see if I could cope. These were desperate days. I was desperate to take them home and yet worried that they weren't getting enough. I didn't do much else but feed day and night.'*

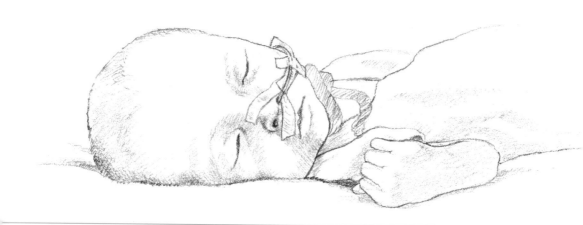

Every time Anna visited SCBU, two floors up, she put her baby to the breast: '*The nurses tried to be helpful but weren't really. They were most interested in giving her a measured quantity of milk. This was expressed breast milk (some of it mine) for the first four days, then the bank was low, so as the healthiest baby on the unit, she had to go on to formula. I was getting a miserable 10ml painfully out with the pump. I was in agony with my cae-sarean wound and the after-pains. I asked for her naso-gastric tube to be left in longer and not to be given bottles in the hope that I would establish feeding at the breast before she got too interested in the bottle teat.*'

Susan found that expressing was vital: '*Karen started breastfeeding once a day by week two and it increased gradually until she was feeding with me all day and on bottles of expressed milk at night until she was able to come home in week seven. My supply was greater than her needs at this stage as I had continued to express whilst feeding her during the day.*'

An encouraging SCBU sister helped Vanessa to make the longed-for contact with her premature son: '*After about two and a half weeks, dur-ing one of my once-daily cuddles with Thomas, an SCBU sister suggested putting him to my breast – it was as if I needed permission to do this; hospi-tal had temporarily robbed me of my motherhood and I wondered why I had not thought to do this before now. I was thrilled at the prospect; my breasts would at long last come into contact with the little mouth that needed me to feed it. I was lucky that the sister was not too busy that day. She demonstrat-ed how I should position Thomas at the breast. Once there Thomas didn't exactly suck (I was warned that he was still too weak to suck properly) but he sniffed and toyed with the nipple in his mouth – it was the first time I felt a let down sensation. The sister was most encouraging, saying things like, "Isn't that wonderful – look he knows what to do what a good little fellow" – I remember glowing with pride.*'

Even having more than one premature baby can become less daunting with help and support, as Simone describes: '*I tried breastfeeding the babies when they were ten days old and to my amazement they all (four quads) man-aged to feed a little, despite their tiny birth weights (ranging from 3lb to 4lb).*'

MANY MOTHERS of premature babies leave hospital before their babies. This adds to the complications involved in expressing milk for the baby. It now has to be transported to the hospital, and journeys to and from the special care unit add to the stresses on the new mother. You may be able to hire an electric breast pump from the hospital; or you can hire Egnell Ameda pumps via the NCT hire scheme. To meet the baby's needs, pumping must be done at the same intervals as a baby would feed. This involves having access to a pump at home and in hospital, and having adequate storage for the expressed milk, until it can be taken to the baby. Many mothers are able to sustain a milk supply by means of the pump, and offering their babies breast-feeds during their visits to hospital. They often feel that it is the most important contribution they can make to their premature baby's care, and that it helps to foster a bond between mother and baby.

Simone's babies remained in hospital for about a month, and she travelled in with her expressed breast milk, having hired an Egnell Ameda electric breast pump from the NCT: *'After ten days the babies were mainly bottle-fed and only had small feeds from me when I could manage it.*

I use the breast pump, which has dual cups, between six and ten times a day, depending on the degree of help I have each day and my level of tiredness. It takes me about 15 minutes to express between 6 and 16fl oz, depending on the time of day, the amount of fluid/food intake I've managed and again, my degree of tiredness.

Despite it being a rather boring task, and very tiring, I have persevered using the breast pump, knowing that the babies have had between a quarter and two-thirds of their feeds from me. I am convinced that it has been a contributory factor in the continued good health of our babies. It has also allowed me several 15-minute solitary breaks every day.

Although a breast pump is expensive to hire, it is a small price to pay for the invaluable breast milk you can give your baby, and it also saves on buying formula milk.'

ONCE YOUR baby is strong enough to feed from the breast, it is beneficial to do so at frequent intervals. For some, there may be a conflict between offering the breast in order to increase supply, and maintaining a record of the baby's intake, as Vanessa describes: *'When I tried to incorporate breastfeeds during my hospital visits it was a problem for the SCBU staff, who are used to measuring fluid intakes to assess growth and development. They would ask me how much milk he had taken – how did I know?'*

YOU MAY find it hard to trust that your body is supplying enough nourishment for your baby once you can no longer see the milk flowing into the pump. Very small babies may have more difficulty in getting a good latch, and skilled help at this stage is vital.

Vanessa found that she could latch Tony on with a little help: *'As Tony progressed from the "hot" to the "cold" nursery, we tried to master breast-feeding together (hoping to cut out the formula feeds). Tony was still small and had trouble latching on. One nurse suggested a nipple shield, whilst another expressed her concern about using one. Heeding the cautionary words about nipple shield dependence, I would remove the shield as soon as the nipple was drawn out; Tony was then able to latch on directly. I used this method for about five days. Tony and I continued to breastfeed (albeit with complementary bottle-feeds) until he was over nine months old.'*

For some mothers, like Frances, sadly, the struggle is just too great: *'I was encouraged to breastfeed (29-week-old two and a half pound baby) and used an electric pump while she was in hospital. She had trouble learning to feed, but eventually managed with a nipple shield. My milk supply never built up enough. I did everything I could to carry on. As she didn't gain weight for two weeks or more I was advised to supplement, but still to breast-feed too – the worst of all worlds as she needed extra at every feed. After five months, she began to refuse the breast and I gave up with relief.'*

WHEN THE day comes to take your premature baby home, you may find that you are suddenly unsure whether you can cope without the support of the special care unit, where you may have built good supportive relationships with the staff. At home, visits from your community midwife and health visitor, although they may be more frequent to begin with, are no substitute for 'on the spot' help and advice. Sometimes, it can seem as if these new helpers are not on the same wavelength, but sometimes they can be the prop which sustains you against those around you who doubt your ability to provide milk for your baby.

Belinda relied on her husband and health visitor to give her the confidence she needed to carry on: *'During the first months at home Karen fed very frequently such that I often heard comments from friends or family members to put her on the bottle: "Surely you haven't got any milk left now."*

These undermined my confidence and I needed a lot of encouragement to ignore them and believe in myself. Nigel was tremendous at this and my health visitor too helped me through one bad patch by suggesting that I thought things over for a few days before coming to any decision – that helped put things in perspective. Looking back at Karen's first months I think I encountered many situations that new mothers do, but, as Karen was chronologically older once she came to these stages I often became over-anxious in case it was a sign that things were not progressing normally.'

Babies who are ill or have special needs

IT IS very distressing to discover that your new baby may be unwell, and unless you have already had experience of breastfeeding, thinking about beginning to express can seem like an added complication at a difficult time for you.

The special care baby unit may be some distance from the maternity wards, and some mothers, who may have just experienced a traumatic delivery, find that they have the added stress of being separated from their baby. If the baby is not premature, and your condition allows, breastfeeding may be possible sooner than with a premature baby. All the special benefits of breast milk will be especially valuable for a baby who has other challenges to face in his new life.

Sometimes, though, feeding may be restricted and breastfeeding may be delayed until the baby's condition improves, as with Gemma's baby: *'After her birth she did not want to feed, which was very unsettling for me. Her sisters had fed soon after birth and I had a bad feeling when she wasn't interested. She kept changing colour and was eventually diagnosed as a "grunting" baby. At an hour she was whisked away to the special nursery where she spent six days. For the first four days she was fed 100% by intravenous drips and was surrounded by wires and monitors. I was only allowed to touch her through the access holes in the incubator. My first visit to the nursery was extremely emotional and traumatic.*

I was determined to start expressing as soon as possible. It was extremely therapeutic to be doing something practical to help. At four days they started with tube feeds, then a day and a half later I was told I could feed her myself. She latched on as if she had been feeding from day one – it was a wonderful moment. The next 24 hours were frustrating as they insisted on test weighing which I found to be terribly inaccurate and every feed was topped up with a tube feed. She had also to be fed four-hourly so when I appeared, she was still full and sleepy from her last feed, didn't take a lot, had to be topped up with a tube, and so it went on. With support from my ward staff, I pushed the nursery staff to put her on demand feeding – eventually they agreed, but on condition she stayed with them. This meant a bit of a sprint as we were at opposite ends of the hospital! I was also still recuperating from my third section – but this was the furthest thing from my mind at this point. However after only two feeds she was allowed up to the ward at 10.30pm one night. It felt like having her all over again!'

Celia thought everything was going perfectly, but then her baby began to be ill: *'Rebecca was born at home in an ideal birth, four to five hours with no complications, no pain relief and a very serene setting. She was put to the breast almost immediately and sucked away contentedly for over half an hour. Everything was wonderful and I felt on top of the world. As she was born at 2.30am we all dozed until the morning.*

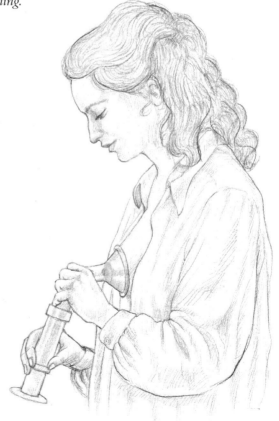

At 7am she started to be ill and the doctor was called. We were sent to hospital and Rebecca was put in special care. I insisted on breastfeeding her that day but by the evening was exhausted and they bottle-fed her in the night. Rebecca was allowed out of special care the following day and I fed her during the day. She started to be ill again that night and was readmitted to special care. Eventually they decided she had meningitis and all feeding stopped as she was on restricted fluids. That day my milk came and my breasts were enormous, hot and sore. I went on the electric pump and froze the expressed milk wondering if Rebecca would live to drink it. For the next two days I pumped every four hours and built up a small collection of frozen milk.

Then Rebecca was on the mend, and she was sucking madly. The doctors said I could feed her once a day. What bliss! She fed

BACKGROUND NOTES

Cleft lip and/or palate

Breastfeeding is likely to be more difficult for a baby with a cleft lip or palate, as it can be harder for him to maintain the seal required between mouth and breast. Even if a baby with a severe cleft is unable to breastfeed, he will still benefit greatly from being fed breast milk. Babies with clefts are prone to ear infections, due to the higher chance of liquid filling the Eustachian tubes (which lead from the back of the nose to the inner ear) when the baby swallows. Breastfed babies with clefts have 75% fewer ear infections and infections of the upper respiratory tract than artificially fed babies, due to the immunological properties of breast milk. Breast milk, being a natural bodily fluid, will not irritate the mucous membranes if it ends up in the 'wrong place'.

Breastfeeding is an important factor in improving the strength of the facial muscles, which will aid the normal development of the baby's face, and may also help the development of normal speech. This is because of the effort involved in obtaining a breastfeed: exercising tongue and gums in a quite specific way.

The position of the cleft will dictate the position that the baby needs to be in, in order to make a seal to allow feeding to begin. A cleft in the soft or hard palate can make it more difficult for a mother to position her baby at the breast so that the breast will be stripped effectively of milk. The baby needs to be able to squeeze the nipple and breast tissue against the roof of his mouth, pressing on the reservoirs of milk. If the cleft is large, this may not be possible. Milk may also leak into the nasal passages, which can cause choking. A dental plate may be made to cover the cleft, which can help. Consult your dentist to find out more. Breasts are soft and can mould to the required shape much more easily than bottles and teats. With a cleft lip, sometimes it only needs the addition of the mother's thumb to cover any remaining gap between breast and mouth for the baby to be able to feed effectively. Often, babies with clefts swallow more air than other breastfed babies, and winding may be necessary during a feed.

Surgery

Treatment for a cleft lip or palate will begin in the first few months of life. Repairs to the lip are usually done quite early, and repairs to the palate are usually carried out at six months to two years of age. Surgeons differ in their opinions about when breastfeeding can recommence after a repair operation. There are several different ways to feed a baby who cannot breastfeed temporarily after his operation, and most hospitals can give guidance about this.

Special guidance

The Cleft Lip and Palate Association (CLAPA) gives practical help and guidance for parents, and support and reassurance to guide them through their difficulties. Several helpful leaflets are also available, including *Help with Feeding*.

CLAPA, 134 Buckingham Palace Road, London SW1. Tel. 0171 824 8110.

beautifully and relaxed afterwards. I determined that if she lived I would breastfeed her whatever the problems.

For the next few days I fed her when allowed and pumped the rest of the time. Gradually I was feeding her completely. Then I got sore, cracked and bleeding nipples. What agony! Still I was going to give her the best, she needed any immunity I could give her in my breast milk and this thought kept me going.

After 10 days I had to go home and leave Rebecca in hospital. I hired an electric pump to pump milk in the night. I was able to get to the hospital for 7am and fed her all day until 6pm. I then pumped milk in the evening and at 1.30 in the morning to take in for her for the following night. The night nurses were great and fed her with my expressed breastmilk and used the frozen supplies when she required more than I could supply. When the frozen supplies were used up they topped up the fresh expressed breast milk with formula.

After 17 days in hospital Rebecca came home. I started feeding her continuously then and found it very, very difficult. I got very sore.'

Holly's baby Joe was diagnosed as having clicky hips and was put into a splint. Although the splint was cumbersome, she thought it should not cause any problems: *'Feeding from my left breast was fine but for some unknown reason he would not latch on to my right breast. I was advised by the midwife in the hospital to hold him under my arm with his legs behind me. This worked, except I didn't find it very comfortable, it was harder to feed discreetly and unless I was in my own house with pillows for him to lie on the problems were getting worse. As he got heavier and his legs got longer, still in a frog position from the splint, I was becoming a little frustrated. He was still feeding fine from the left and I kept putting him across me on the right but he still would not latch on. Feeding would last between an hour and an hour and a half and it seemed to be about every three hours. It was hard work.*

Eventually the cause was found. At his eight-week hip check he was diagnosed as having a wry neck (torticollis). This is where the neck muscle is stretched and then contracts and his head constantly fell to the side. He started physiotherapy immediately, but by the time his neck problem was cured and his splint was removed he had put on so little weight that I was advised to top up with bottle milk and by five months I had dried up completely.'

FOR SOME mothers, like Mina, despite their determination, their baby's condition does not allow them to breastfeed: *'When my son was*

FEEDING FILE

Positions for feeding a baby with a cleft

Feeding may take much longer than normal, and patient experimentation will pay dividends. A rather more upright position than normal is often better for the baby, as it helps prevent milk from leaking into the nasal passages. No matter what position you decide is best, stick to the general rule of ensuring that your baby is facing you, with his head and neck in line and not twisting round, which makes swallowing difficult.

Straddie position

Sit your baby in your lap, facing you, with his legs one either side of your stomach. You may need to sit him on pillows to bring him up to the level of your breast. You can then see where to position your nipple so that he can get the best latch. It can help to tilt the baby's head back slightly as he latches on. You are then free to use your other hand to help the baby to make a seal between his mouth and your breast, or just to support his chin.

Football hold

The football hold described in Chapter Seven can be modified to suit the baby's needs. Again, pillows may be needed to raise the baby up to the level of your breast. Position your baby so that he is sitting up beside you, facing you, with his legs and feet under your arm. Support your baby with your arm, and his head gently in your hand. You may need to support your breast with your other hand to help the baby to make a seal.

Preference for one side

Due to the position of the cleft, some babies may have a strong preference for feeding in one position, and swapping sides may be difficult. It may be easier for you to keep the baby in his preferred position, and simply slide him across to the other breast. Or you could just feed him from one breast.

---

born prematurely, I was determined to breastfeed. I hadn't even bought a bottle or steriliser! In the event he couldn't breastfeed or bottle-feed. He was born with a very severe bilateral cleft lip and palate and the only way I could get milk inside him, with a struggle, was to spoon-feed.'

Breastfeeding on a children's ward

IT CAN BE difficult for you as a breastfeeding mother if your baby needs admission to a children's ward where staff may lack training and time to help with breastfeeding, or the regime is not pro-breastfeeding. There is no certainty that anyone on a children's ward will be knowledgeable and up-to-date about breastfeeding.

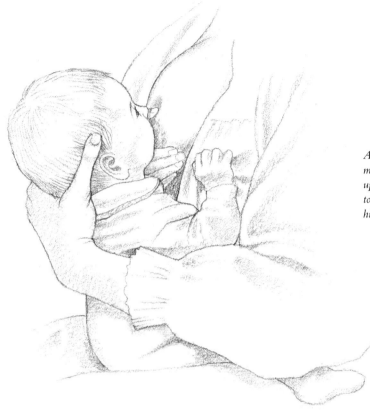

A baby with a cleft lip or palate may feed more easily in an upright position. Use your hand to help him form a seal between his mouth and your breast.

At five weeks old, Rose's baby had a severe attack of croup and they were admitted to the local hospital: *'He made an amazing noise as he crouped and screamed simultaneously so the consultant couldn't hear a thing when he tried to examine him. I suggested letting him suck to calm him down which the consultant thought a good idea. However the look I got from the ward sister will always stay with me. As soon as the ward round was over she sent a porter in to our isolation cubicle with screens and read me the riot act about feeding behind these in case someone walked through the ward, and stopping to look in at us, saw me feeding a baby! I felt more isolated than ever.*

The maternity unit in the hospital had an amazing lady known as the lactation sister who promoted breastfeeding on the maternity wards. The consultants called for her to watch me feed and prove me competent. I felt, as she watched, that my rate of flow was being calibrated. However, it was a relief to have her confirm my opinion as to the amount that he was taking even if she did criticise my droopy breasts!

One of the more junior doctors worried that he had no record of the volume that the baby was receiving and one suggested that they needed a drip just because he was breastfed in case he became dehydrated. The nursing staff insisted that we fill in a chart that stated how long he fed for and wouldn't consider that my estimate of how much he was taking might be more useful. I began to wish that my breasts were calibrated like measuring cylinders. I was constantly criticised by the nursing staff for feeding him on demand. My theory was that if he had enough energy to try to feed and breathe then I wanted him to receive some nourishment. However, all the other children on the ward were fed strictly four-hourly. I was fortunate to receive support from my mother, who had been a midwife in the days when not to breastfeed a baby was an abnormality that had to be recorded on a midwife's register.

As Patrick held his own and began to recover, the consultants then began to take me to task about feeding on demand. I was told that feeding more often than every four hours exhausted the mother and deprived the rest of my family. I pointed out that as the mother of a less than two-year-old and a baby who could rarely sleep for more than an hour before his breathing trouble woke him, I was quite pleased to be able to sit down every couple of hours, have a drink, read to my toddler and suckle my baby.'

Admission to a children's ward can be even more difficult if facilities for mothers are also limited. Finding enough food to satisfy a breastfeeding mother's appetite may be a problem. Lena felt that her needs were not taken into consideration at all: *'My daughter was transferred to a children's hospital at birth and I elected to go with her to breastfeed and closely follow her progress. Care obviously is for the babies but newly-delivered mothers need care too, especially at a traumatic time. The lack of a bed was probably the worst thing as a lie-down during the day was impossible. A zed-bed at night was available in the coffee cupboard and so postnatal exercises were difficult to do, privacy for examinations minimal and rest impossible. Facilities were minimal, loos in a different block, canteen far away and one filthy bath. Breastfeeding advice and support was not available as the staff had no experience or training in this. Nurses with children themselves were of more help, but many younger nurses didn't know what to do when confronted with a tearful mum with her difficulties in feeding.'*

Babies with special needs who are able to feed at the breast will gain comfort from the contact, apart from the benefit of breast milk.

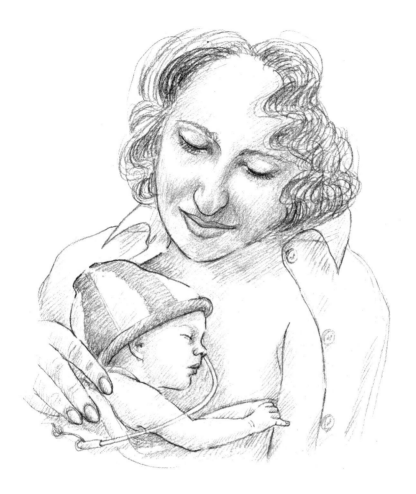

Breastfeeding may also help you to bond with your baby. Supplying milk for your baby may be the only thing which you can do to help the medical staff to care for him. Chloe needed to feel close to her son, given the seriousness of his condition: *'Breastfeeding my baby with his uncertain diagnosis was the most comforting thing for both of us. We remained close and untouched by the seemingly disastrous events. Even when his echocardiogram (ultrasound of the heart) showed that our second son indeed had a large congenital heart defect (40% of children with Down's syndrome have) I was not put off from feeding him. The specialists said he would not gain weight rapidly and could require supplemental feedings. We were required to return him for regular weight checks and blood tests for a period after his discharge from hospital. By the time the diagnosis of Down's syndrome had been confirmed we were fairly convinced though we still prayed it should not be true. Thus our start*

together was a bumpy one but never did we find breastfeeding to be a problem. It was the one joy I had planned for that no one could take away!'

When Gail's second son Phillip was only two days old, he was found to be suffering from a major heart defect and was admitted to hospital. He underwent a minor operation that night, to stabilise his condition, then had to wait a week before the open heart surgery to correct the problem could be performed: *'I had successfully breastfed my elder son for almost a year, and was anxious to do the same for Phillip. It was especially important for me, at a time when so much depended on the skills and experience of the surgical and medical staff, to feel that there was at least one thing I could do to give him the best possible chance of coming through the operation.*

Luckily, the hospital was able to accommodate me in a room in the same building as the children's ward, so that the nursing staff could call me down for night-time feeds; and Phillip fed so successfully that he'd regained his birth weight after only five days.

A couple of days before the operations I started to practise expressing milk with an electric pump, in a rather poky, though adequate, room close to the ward. The results were frozen in small volumes for later use. Then, during the time that Phillip was in intensive care, I expressed three times a day, in order to produce about 6oz at each session.

After the first day in intensive care, Phillip was allowed to receive steadily increasing amounts of my expressed milk through a naso-gastric tube. Once again, it was very satisfying to feel that I was contributing my own share to his recovery. On the evening of the second day after the operation, Phillip was taken off the ventilator, and I was able to give him a small breastfeed – an experience which I felt we'd both been missing!

Over the next couple of days, as Phillip's fluid intake still had to be limited, I breastfed him "restrictively": that is, he was not actively encouraged to feed, nor to return to the breast if he came off. After that, we were able to return to normal demand feeding.'

Sometimes you may find that, when an older baby who is still having breastfeeds falls ill, maintaining your supply becomes a lifeline for you. When Chloe's son, Tom, was 11 months old she suffered a very frightening experience: *'Tom had been suffering from a cold and had been very needy, wanting to be at the breast all the time. I was very sore and gave* him to dad – *he finally fell asleep. When he awoke he was crying and distressed. I cleared his nose and put him on my shoulder to take him downstairs to feed but when I placed him across my lap I noticed he was staring with both eyes towards the left. He could not suck at my breast. He could not move his right arm or leg. He had experienced a stroke.*

After seven days on a respirator, and ten days in the intensive therapy unit, the doctors questioned his survival. My milk supply diminished to nil. Although I was hearing that there may be no baby to give my milk to, I felt it was once more the bond which kept us united. I arranged to use the electric pump. So I began with half an ounce and built up to three to four ounces. It somehow helped to keep me going and divert my energy from pity to hope. Once Tom came off the respirator and tube feedings were begun it was my milk that was offered and supplemented by soymilk. Oh joy of joys when Tom was released to the children's ward and he turned to breastfeed. I had not been sure that it would ever happen! He was truly determined, and I was forever grateful that I had not given up totally.'

MOTHERS WITH SPECIAL NEEDS

IF YOU have a disability or become ill, you may need special help with breastfeeding. Sometimes, your carers may feel that breastfeeding is only adding to the strain on your system, but you may want to continue to breastfeed. Sensitivity on the part of carers will help you to come to terms with your loss if you have to stop. In many cases, with diagnosis and treatment, breastfeeding can continue.

Sylvia had a brain operation for an aneurism (a weak blood vessel) which resulted in loss of some neurological function and consequent weakness on her right side: *'I have very little effective use of my right arm and I find it difficult to walk, although this is somewhat improved when I wear an electronic stimulator. My son was two at the time and since then I have had a daughter. Breastfeeding my son was a lovely experience and I wanted to breastfeed my daughter. The advantages of breastfeeding have all applied, but more so in my case as it meant that the difficulties of preparing and handling feed bottles with one hand were removed.*

Naturally I anticipated more problems breastfeeding my daughter than I had with my son, but I found that they could all be dealt with. For example, I was able to cope with the difficulty of holding the baby while she fed by using pillows. I was able to acquire a V-shaped pillow which was ideal in providing secure support. Having breastfed before my loss of arm and leg function, I realised that most of the problems I experienced were what any mother would be faced with whether disabled or not.'

Not only was Helen's son diagnosed as allergic to formula milk, but he also had a medical problem. Breastfeeding, indeed any type of feeding, became increasingly difficult and then Helen discovered she was ill: *'I suddenly started losing dramatic amounts of weight (without trying) and was finally referred to a specialist. I was diagnosed as having coeliac disease. This is a condition often referred to as gluten allergy (though it is not really an allergy). A coeliac is unable to absorb vitamins and minerals properly – hence a fairly small baby and quite simply a lack of resources enabling*

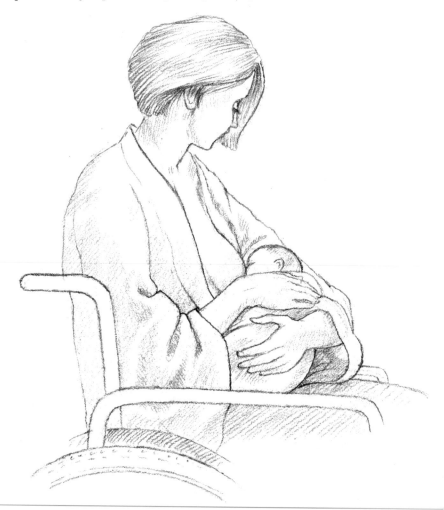

establishment of a good milk supply. As soon as I started a gluten-free diet I began to feel better and finally had a reason for my failure to breastfeed.

I am now considered perfectly healthy (and glad to report my son's good health). However, I still regret not being able to give my son the very best start in life, but I can be happy that I did all possible under the circumstances. I am informed that as a diagnosed coeliac following a strict diet, I should be able to fully breastfeed any additions to the family.'

Sudden illness striking can mean a disruption to breastfeeding. If your milk supply is well established, it need not spell the end of breastfeeding, though. If you need to be admitted to hospital, you should be able to take your fully breastfed baby with you. Norma found that frequent breastfeeds helped her supply to recover: *'When Sarah was about three months old, I caught a horrible tummy bug which meant I didn't eat for several days and for two days I couldn't keep down water. My doctor called in, poked my breasts and laughed, "Ha! Empty! Get a tin of SMA, your breastfeeding days are over!" I ignored her advice, let Sarah suckle often and gave her a little boiled water from a spoon as I was worried she'd dehydrate. My milk soon returned when I could keep water down.'*

BREASTFEEDING may have particular practical advantages for you.

Claudette suffers from chronic asthma: *'As to my chest problem: pregnancy was good for my asthma (although I was still on high doses of inhaled steroids and had to have one course of steroid tablets) but now my asthma is worsening again. As well as helping to protect Emma from asthma and eczema, I have found breastfeeding to be helpful to me. The convenience, especially at night, is a real bonus. I am often breathless at night when I feed her, but all I have to do is take a few puffs of my reliever inhaler and I can immediately feed her. I make life even easier for myself by having Emma sleep in*

BACKGROUND NOTES

ParentAbility

ParentAbility, the NCT's network for parents with disabilities, provides mutual support during pregnancy and parenthood. The NCT also has a national 'Special Situations Register', listing the names of parents who have experienced special situations and who are happy to be contacted by others in a similar position. Some NCT branches also have local registers. For further details, contact:

> ParentAbility
> The National Childbirth Trust
> Alexandra House
> Oldham Terrace
> Acton
> London W3 6NH.
>
> Tel: 0181 992 8637.

bed with me so I don't even have to get up. The weight of the baby on my chest can be a problem, but I can support her on a pillow on my lap, which greatly reduces the pressure on my chest (I wanted to feed her lying down, but that has not proved possible as I cannot breathe well lying on my side). Sometimes I get a sore nipple when I cough, throwing Emma off my breast rather violently, but Emma seems to take this in her stride and the soreness is short-lived. Bottle-feeding at night would be difficult, as I would have to actually get up and do things. The other advantage of breastfeeding is that the prolactin hormone you produce when feeding relaxes you – always a bonus to an asthmatic as you need less oxygen when you are relaxed and tension can make the wheezing worse. Obviously, I don't need to carry the bottle-feeding paraphernalia around, like sterile water, powder and bottles and the less I need to carry the better, because it can be impossible to carry things when I am breathless.'

SOMETIMES IT may take time and ingenuity to find the best solution to practical difficulties.

Libby has had ME for nearly 11 years. During that time she has had two babies and has breastfed both. ME affects the muscles and brain. Her main symptoms are fatigue, muscle pain and weakness, memory problems and feeling exceptionally cold: *'With the first baby it was difficult to get comfortable, the baby felt heavy – it was a strain and the night feeds meant I got very cold. With the second I did better in every respect, although the second pregnancy had made my ME very much worse. This time, though, I knew how to breastfeed and found ways of overcoming the ME problems. I lay on the bed with the baby's weight on my body (I had tried to sit holding the first one). That solved the weight/muscle problems. I had the baby by the side of me at night (the first one had been in a separate room) so this avoided either of us becoming cold.'*

Isla's right hand is affected by cerebral palsy: *'I am unable to manipulate my fingers of that hand. This caused problems when breastfeeding, and so my one-day-old baby son and I had to experiment with different positions and pillows until we found a way which suited us. It was only a small problem, but it seemed a very large one at the time, and I did feel very lonely because the nurses in the hospital either could not understand the problem or did not have the time to help me solve it. I wanted to find a solution quickly, not weeks after giving birth. I had my daughter when my son was under two years of age, and so I had my hands full. I really do believe that there is an answer to everything provided you have a bit of imagination.'*

Gillian was consigned to bed for six weeks, because of a back problem, when her son Francis was two weeks old: *'I'd fed Francis lying down before, in hospital and at home, but now I had two slipped discs and it all got fairly tricky. Feeding now involved lying on my side while getting Francis in position and latched on with one hand; and holding a breast shell in the cup of my nursing bra with the other (nursing bras are designed to support a non-feeding breast when the owner is vertical, not when she is lying on her side). When he'd finished the first side, I'd have to go through some very difficult manoeuvres to turn me and him over, rearrange the drip-spotted muslin we were lying on, and start the whole caper again on side two. Still, it was definitely worth it: I couldn't do anything else for Francis at this time, or for myself, and since this appeared to be the single part of motherhood at which I excelled, I was pretty determined to hang on to it.'*

Extra help with household tasks and caring for other children may be vital for you if you need extra rest to maintain your milk supply. If this doesn't happen, you may feel as Cheryl did: *'The main problem this time was that as I was so tired I couldn't keep up with the demand and I couldn't rest enough to improve it. I had an older child to consider. I didn't have the energy to keep feeding my baby more frequently because it then left little or no time for rest/sleep.'*

The psychological benefits of breastfeeding are also important. Janie explains why it is important to her: *'Because of my disability (I have multiple sclerosis and use a wheelchair when I go out), I feel I have to prove I can cope better than everyone else just so people don't think I'm helpless. I think breastfeeding Hannah helped in that respect because people could see she was really my baby and she was growing and thriving because of the milk I was giving her.'*

SHOULD YOU suffer from postnatal depression, you may find, as these mothers did, that breastfeeding is an important way of building your self-confidence at a time when feelings of inadequacy may be strong.

'*Despite suffering from postnatal depression after the birth of my first baby I found great comfort in my ability to breastfeed. I did not feel that my mothering skills were very good but at least my growing baby enabled me to see that at least one aspect of motherhood I had got right.*'

'*My main symptom was extreme tiredness. I found it almost impossible to get up and dressed, let alone do housework or shop. I don't think I would ever have managed to prepare bottles. Lying in bed feeding Sara was about all I could manage.*'

Breastfeeding after breast surgery

IF YOU have had any kind of breast surgery before having children, you may wonder, like Morag, whether you will be able to breastfeed: '*When I was 19, I had a benign lump removed from my right breast. At the time, the only thought that occurred to me was whether the lump was malignant or not. However, at 26 I was expecting our first baby – the wish to breastfeed was strong and I began to wonder whether I would have any problems due to the operation, as the scar is pretty inflexible.*

Ruth was born and fed well from both sides until by five or six months and on to pureed food she gave up feeding from the right breast – I presumed because as I had dropped one feed and she slept through, the milk supply was dwindling. I continued to feed her from the left side until she was eleven months.

When Libby, our second daughter, was born she gave up on the right breast after only a couple of weeks. However with the advice that "twins manage on one" ringing in my ears, I continued to feed her until eleven months, just from the one side.'

IT WOULD be fair to say that your ability to breastfeed will probably depend on the surgery which you have had done and how long ago it was performed. A simple 'lumpectomy', as Morag describes, is not likely to damage the breast enough to prevent all milk production. She found that the breast which had undergone surgery did not seem to produce as much milk, but this is not always the case. Your surgeon is probably the best person to discuss the likelihood of success with. He should be able to tell you whether he had to cut through any of the milk ducts. If you can still feel sensation in your nipples, this will make breastfeeding easier for you, as it means that you do not have much damage to your nerves. You may feel that, even if you cannot produce all the milk which your baby needs, it will be worth breast-feeding anyway. You could talk through your feelings about this with a breastfeeding counsellor.

If you have had cosmetic surgery – augmentation or reduction – you may still be able to breastfeed. Again, this will depend on how much damage was done to the structure of the ducts during the oper-ation. Silicone bags inserted behind the breast tissue, to enlarge the breasts, are less likely to interfere with breastfeeding, although you may feel more uncomfortable initially when your milk comes in. A reduction operation may be more problematic if the nipple has been resited, which is likely to have involved severing the ducts. Sometimes, the ducts will join back together, but this is unpre-dictable. Once again, your surgeon will be the best person to give you advice on the possibilities for you.

If only one breast has had surgery, you will in any case be able to breastfeed successfully from the other.

THE ADVANTAGES of breastfeeding are particularly marked for moth-ers and babies with special needs. For the babies, breastfeeding offers comfort and health benefits. For you, there are practical advantages and the boost to morale which successful breastfeeding brings. Both you and your baby require the best possible help and support to estab-lish breastfeeding, taking account of your individual circumstances and needs.

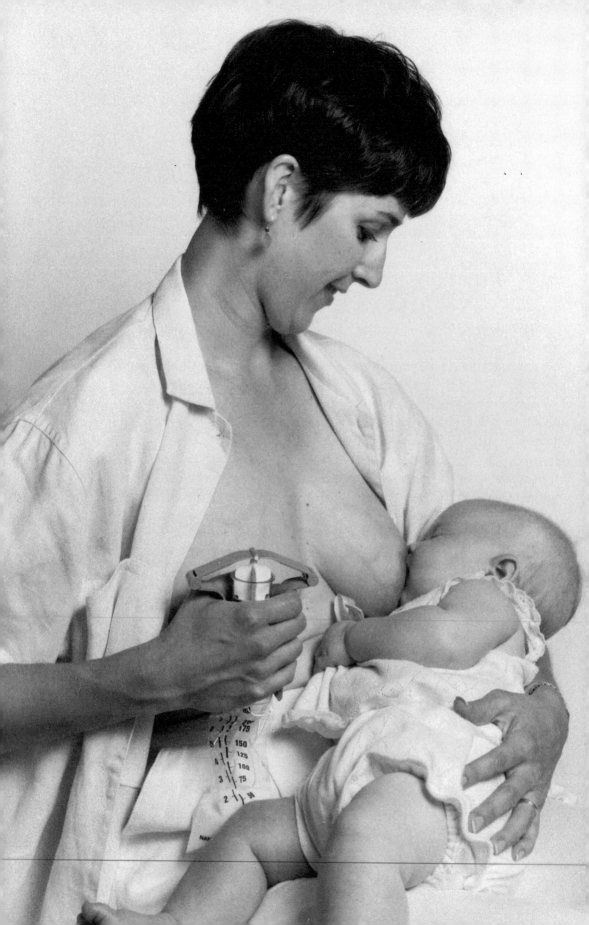

CHAPTER *eleven* Breastfeeding and returning to work

IT HAS BECOME fairly common for women to return to paid work within a few months of the birth of their baby. There may be financial pressures to return, or concerns about career progress if you are away for long, or it may be by choice. Those who are entitled to better than the basic maternity pay and leave may not return to work so soon. However, many mothers return after the 14 weeks' maternity leave to which all women are now entitled, or sooner, depending on their circumstances.

There is little recent evidence about the effect of returning to work on breastfeeding. Does an early return to work deter mothers from starting to breastfeed, or influence how long they feed for? A study of mothers in 1990 found that mothers of first babies who were working tended, if anything, to be more likely to breastfeed than those who were not working. It also found no evidence that returning to work significantly shortened the length of time for which a mother breastfed.[1] Whether such findings will remain true as more mothers of young babies go back to work, remains to be seen.

Natalie made arrangements at work that enabled her to be with her baby for as long as possible: *'I took the maximum maternity leave from work (paid and unpaid) and then arranged with my employer to take my outstanding annual leave at the rate of two and a half days a week. This effectively entitled me to seven months off and then to three months of part-time work, before going back full time. Because of this long maternity leave I always planned to breastfeed Esther and to continue with a morning and evening feed as long as she demanded it.'*

For Mandy, who returned to work sooner, the choice was more difficult: *'I felt pressurised to bottle-feed because I knew from the outset that I would be returning to work when my son was eight weeks old. In the event he was totally breastfed until I returned to work, at which stage bottles of for-mula quickly took over. I was surprised how much this upset me.'*

FEELINGS ABOUT RETURNING TO WORK

RETURNING TO work may bring a range of different feelings. If you have had some choice about the length of your maternity leave, you may feel ready to return, although the wrench of leaving your baby may still be strong. Or you may feel angry, sad or guilty about having to return.

When the time came for Peggy to go back to work, she felt ready: *'Of course I missed her, but I knew she was in good hands. She still had early morning and night-time feeds, which became especially important times for me. I think that we both benefited from being apart from one another. She got the stimulation and variety of other people, who had time and energy for her. I got the opportunity to engross myself in a satisfying job and came back fresh to her at the end of the day.'*

Lois felt nowhere near ready to return to work after four months when she said she'd first go part time: *'I was feeding every three hours or so and Tessa wouldn't take a bottle. I wanted to carry on breastfeeding but saw no practical way to combine it with the demands of work. I had not yet come to terms with motherhood and felt it necessary to be there all the time to be any good at it. My new manager didn't understand and saw my indecision as lack of commitment. I resigned, feeling that my "perfect" mother should always be there for her children. Part of me was glad to lose the pressure of work, but part wasn't. My resentment at having to stay at home made me more tense and Tessa felt this.'*

Tessa felt that returning to work altered the focus of her relationship with her son: *'Because only I could feed and nurture him I felt a huge sense of responsibility and an enormous wrench at leaving him. Financially, we had no choice but I did not know beforehand how I was going to feel once he was born. I felt that going back to work definitely damaged the closeness and inten-sity of our relationship and this really upset me. I also felt very guilty and this made me all the more determined to succeed with breastfeeding – I felt at least it was something I could do for my baby.'*

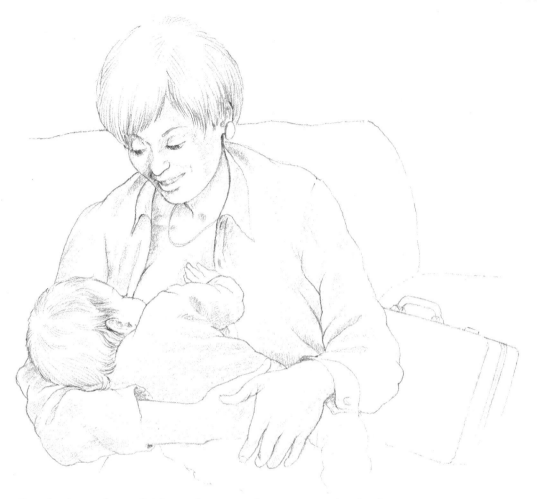

Continuing to breastfeed may be a way for you to maintain the special bond which you have with your baby – this is how Danielle and Barbara felt: *'When I finally went back to work I felt the breastfeeding was a part of the bond I did not want to break. I fed up until the last minute before going to work and expressed during the day.'*

'Apart from feeling as though I was giving my daughter the best start in life, breastfeeding has given us a special closeness, which as a mum who had to return to work very early on was an extremely important feeling for me. It has enabled our relationship to be special; I am after all sharing something with her that no other carer can. I am not saying that mums who don't breastfeed don't feel those special things too, just that, for me, it was important to feel them in that way.'

Paula was not looking forward to her return to work and she was worried how Charlotte would take to a bottle with her childminder: *'I found it reassuring to see my little bags of breast milk filling up the freezer. I think this was my way of trying to come to terms with my anxieties about leaving Charlotte: expressing milk was something positive I could do about a situation I could not fully control.'*

FEEDING: THE OPTIONS

IF YOU ARE breastfeeding, you have a number of options for feeding your baby when you return to work. The choice you make depends on your individual circumstances and feelings. You may decide to give your baby breast milk only, or to use a combination of breast milk and formula milk or other drinks. Or you may decide to wean your baby from the breast. You may find it helpful to discuss these options with a breastfeeding counsellor or other working mothers who have breastfed, to help you choose what will suit you best.

If you decide to give your baby breast milk only, you may express milk to be given to your baby by her carer whilst you are away, and breastfeed when you are at home. Or you may work at home, or be able to visit your baby during the day to breastfeed. Older babies may be taking other drinks and not need breast milk whilst you are at work. You may be very determined to continue breastfeeding, or you may be prepared to stop if difficulties arise.

Mavis was dreading going back to work – having established breast-feeding and seeing her daughter, Rosalyn, thriving on it, she didn't relish the thought of giving up: *'I decided that I would try expressing milk to leave for her to be fed by the childminder. After consulting my health visitor, who was a great support, and various magazines etc., I purchased a hand pump and went to work. The results to begin with were nothing less than discouraging. Eventually I was able to get a fair amount out (6–8oz) and also discovered the optimum times to express.*

I am happy to say that I have now been back to work (part time) for four weeks and expressing is going very well. I have a freezer full of expressed milk that has initially been frozen in ice cube trays and then transferred to freezer bags. The knowledge that I have plenty of "back up" milk in the freezer (enough for two weeks) helps me to relax when I am unable to express the exact amount she needs each week. Every week I arrive on the door of my childminder with Rosalyn and a carrier bag full of frozen breast milk.

My employer is supportive in making space for me to express my milk at work twice a day and letting me store it in the fridge (no one has used it yet for their coffee either). Although expressing does require determination and a great deal of organisation, to me it has been well worth the effort and I will continue for as long as is possible and appropriate.'

Jacqui continued breastfeeding after returning to work part time because she enjoys feeding, it was well established and she didn't feel ready to break the bond: *'On both occasions the wee ones were ten or eleven months old before I returned to work, so I had plenty of opportunity to build up a supply of frozen milk to leave at home. By this stage my milk supply had settled down, and although my breasts were very full at the end of my working day I didn't need to express milk at work. As I only work two days a week I continued to breastfeed at lunchtime on my non-working days without any problems in terms of milk production.'*

By the time Natalie went back to work her daughter, Esther, was ready for a full day at nursery: *'Esther was still taking a midday feed, so for the first couple of weeks back at work I drove over at lunch time and fed Esther at nursery. It was a bit inconvenient but I didn't mind doing it as I felt it got both of us used to the idea of changing our routines gradually. The nursery staff were very supportive and I never felt uncomfortable about sitting breastfeeding there.'*

YOU MAY decide on a combination of breast and formula milk: perhaps breast milk when you are at home, and formula milk whilst you are working. It may be difficult for you to express milk, or you may prefer not to. Once breastfeeding is well established, you may find that your breasts, and your baby, adapt well to a combination of breast milk and formula. You may have problems with leaking or overfull breasts until your supply settles down. You may need to express a small amount of milk at work to ease your discomfort. Pressing on the nipples may help prevent leaking: this can be done discreetly if you cross your arms. It may help to keep a spare top at work for emergencies.

Kelly found that a combination of breast and bottle worked well for her: *'When I returned to work (when my first child was seven months and then when my second child was five months), I was still fully breastfeeding on my days off, but found, although it was a bit uncomfortable at first, that both my body and the babies adapted very quickly to feeding from me on my days off and at morning and night and taking a bottle of formula in my absence from their carers.'*

ANOTHER ALTERNATIVE is to wean your baby from the breast when returning to work, if you are ready to finish breastfeeding or if you feel that working and breastfeeding would not be possible.

Hazel chose to stop breastfeeding when she returned to work: *'I was lucky to be able to negotiate a long maternity break, using maternity leave, then holidays, then study leave – though I didn't do a lot of studying. By the end of this time I felt ready to finish breastfeeding.'*

A job involving long hours away from her baby eventually left Naomi with no choice: *'I continued with the evening feed until she was 17 months and only stopped then because I changed jobs and am now commuting to central London. The vagaries of British Rail, and the need to attend evening meetings mean I could not guarantee to be home to give her an evening feed so I decided it was better for her to have a regular bedtime routine that did not require my presence.'*

IF YOU ARE very keen to breastfeed, you may decide to leave your job because breastfeeding and work do not seem to be compatible.

Danielle's baby more or less led the way: *'The baby would only accept bottles of breast milk from my husband, not the childminder! He became quite weak by starving himself if I wasn't there even though he was on mixed feeding by this time. I gave up work again after a few weeks.'*

Jackie's employer made it clear where she stood: *'I went back to work as a cook when my baby was six weeks old. I wanted to carry on fully breastfeeding but my employer was very unsympathetic. I was not allowed a break to leave my work and feed the baby elsewhere and when I expressed milk at work I was told that the other staff were upset by what I was doing so I must stop. As my work was casual I had no rights, so I left.'*

FEEDING FILE

Expressing milk for your baby: things to consider before you return to work

● Everyone's work situation is different. You may find it useful to talk through your specific conditions with a breastfeeding counsellor and your employer

● Choosing an appropriate pump is important. If possible, try out the various options some time before you return to work

● Some NCT branch newsletters carry 'sales and wants' advertisements. You may find a second-hand pump available

● Introduce your baby to a bottle (or cup) well in advance of your return date. Someone other than you may be better – your baby will expect a breastfeed from you and may not accept a substitute offered by you

● Check out with your baby's carer that she is willing to store and carefully defrost the expressed breast milk left for your baby

● If possible, have a 'trial run' before the first day you must leave your baby. This could highlight any unforeseen difficulties. There may be time to rearrange your plans accordingly.

EXPRESSING MILK

YOU MAY plan to express milk, at home and/or at work, to meet all or most of your baby's demands. You may need to express milk at work for your own comfort, or to keep up your supply. Maintaining a supply of expressed breast milk can be a major commitment, especially if you work full time and have little or no support. Like breastfeeding itself, expressing milk may take practice. Often, it is easier to begin to express milk before you return to work so that you have time to gain experience and to decide what method of expressing suits you best. It also allows you to build up a stock of frozen milk for later use.

Wendy has developed her own particular routine at work: *'I use a breast pump at home, but at work I express by hand, as it is easier for sterilising purposes. I have my own soap and towel and I express into a sterilised milk container, then transfer the milk to a sterilised baby bottle which I keep in a cool bag big enough to contain five ice bricks and the bottle. I also pack the bag with bubbly stuff. It is very important to have a good cool bag and to only open it to top up the milk.'*

BREAST PUMPS

● Breast pumps work by suction which draws the milk out of the breast. The suction is created either by hand or by electric power. The suction strength on most pumps can be adjusted

● Different pumps suit different women

● Some pumps are easier to assemble and clean than others. You may find it useful to talk to someone with experience of pumping to discover these

● If you buy a pump and you find it doesn't work after you have given it a good try, take it back

● Some pumps come supplied with a soft plastic shield, a Flexishield, which fits inside the rigid plastic funnel which is placed over the nipple area. The Flexishield moulds round the breast and when the pump is working, the action emulates a baby sucking. The stimulation of the breast and so the yield of breast milk is greater

● Flexishields are also sold separately. Contact Egnell Ameda or the local NCT pump agent.

Hand Pumps

● A simple hand pump may be sufficient for occasional part-time work. They cost around £15 and are simple to sterilise

● Most hand pumps work by pressure on a lever, or by pulling a cylinder in and out

● Lever pumps are designed for one-handed use, and some women manage to feed their baby at one breast whilst they express from the other

● All hand pumps are small and portable, and quiet to use, so would be suitable for expressing at work

● Some women complain that with frequent use, the plastic parts on hand pumps wear out

● Avoid the hand pump, or 'breast reliever', as it is properly called, which consists of a rubber bulb attached to a plastic funnel which fits over the breast, sometimes with a screw-on bottle attached. It is very difficult to obtain suction by squeezing the bulb and the pump cannot be sterilised properly.

Melanie is a full-time teacher. She found expressing easy first time around: *'It used to take less than 30 seconds to get a let down on the pump, and in the end my childminder and I both threw out frozen reserves. So when it came to Gregor, my second child, I hadn't laid in large advance stocks. It was a nasty shock when in my first week back I found I was only getting 100–120ml per pumping, and Gregor needed two feeds of 200ml plus. I reinstated the midnight feed, took to pumping three times (lunch time, 4pm*

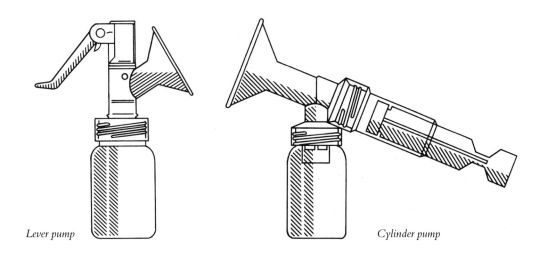

Lever pump   *Cylinder pump*

and 6pm) and actually tried to rest a bit. Five weeks after I started, supply was just about keeping up with demand.'

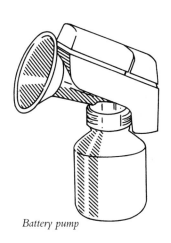

The most important factor when expressing your milk, however you choose to do it, is to ensure that your milk is letting down. This means that you are collecting the fat-rich hindmilk and not just the foremilk stored in the ducts. Melanie discovered this for herself: *'It would appear, even to my untutored eye, that the 50ml or so which can be obtained after half an hour's effort without a let down must be foremilk only, as the cream doesn't rise to the top in the fridge as it does with milk from a satisfactory pumping session.*

Battery pump

The books suggest that you look at a picture of the baby, concentrate your mind on his little downy head and think milk. I have actually found that what has to happen for me is to get so engrossed in the newspaper, or the crossword, or talking to my husband after work, that I don't think about it, and then it will "go".'

Rita sometimes had to encourage her let down: *'If I'm very engorged I have no problems expressing milk, but if I'm having difficulty starting I usually feed the baby on the other side. It can be a bit awkward, trying to support him and express at the same time but it usually works. I've also found standing under a shower usually results in a let down.'*

BREAST PUMPS

Electric pumps

● Electric pumps are powered by battery or mains electricity; some use either

● Pumps range from small, lightweight, hand-held battery pumps to larger electric models weighing around 2.5kg which rest on a table

● Prices vary from about £25 for a small battery pump to around £400 for a large electric pump, plus running costs

● The suction strength varies with the size of the pump, so a small battery pump will not necessarily help you to express more milk than a hand pump, although it may be less tiring

● Batteries run down very quickly with regular use, so buying rechargeable batteries and a charger is a worthwhile investment

● Large electric pumps have attachments for expressing both breasts at once – dual pumping – which is speedier and usually increases the amount obtained

● Electric pumps make some noise

● The Egnell 'Elite' is a new electric pump which is light and easy to use

● Large electric pumps may be hired locally from the National Childbirth Trust and/or La Leche League. Telephone 0181 992 8637 for details of your nearest pump hire agent; or contact Egnell Ameda Ltd, Unit 2, Belvedere Trading Estate, Taunton, Somerset TA1 1BA.

FACILITIES AND support for breastfeeding mothers at the work place vary. It is useful to contact your employer in advance to make sure that there is somewhere where you can express milk at work.

Jinny was particularly fortunate with her employer: *'I decided for many reasons that I wanted to continue breastfeeding after I had to return to work. I felt it was still some part of me that I could give to him even though I couldn't be there with him all day. Since he was now being exposed to more germs and other children, I felt that the antibodies my milk could provide were helping his immune system to develop. And purely selfishly, it was my way of reminding myself and others that even if I was back at work, I was a mum first and foremost.*

I had a wonderful time. Although I worked in a very male oriented profession, as a petroleum engineer in an oilfield, I found my co-workers and superiors to be very supportive. I had a wonderful electric dual breast pump and I

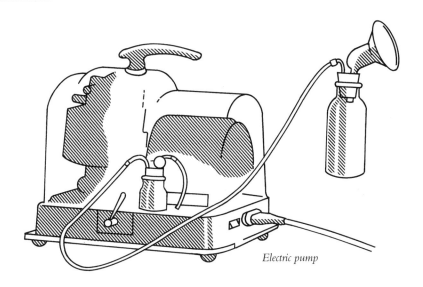

Electric pump

would take 15-minute morning and afternoon breaks and could easily pump 18–22 ounces. I did have a private office, although no lock, and we had a refrigerator/freezer in the coffee bar. I took quite a bit of good-natured ribbing from my co-workers especially over my full breasts right before "milking", as they called it, but I felt in no way offended. They seemed to adopt my son as the department mascot. I found it so relaxing to take those 15-minute breaks, to concentrate just on Josh, to let go of any stress at work and know that I was doing something that I felt was very important.'

Carla had a slightly different, but equally supportive experience: *'I told my direct superior that I wished to have somewhere to go and express my milk. He arranged for me to go to the nurse's room. I express twice a day. I do not use the fridge at work because it might be off-putting for my workmates to open the fridge and find human milk in it. Also, if you keep your milk by your side all day, you are sure not to forget it in the evening. I keep mine in a cool bag underneath my desk.'*

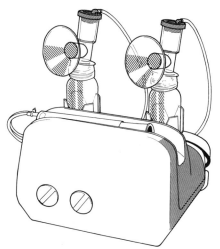

Lightweight electric pump

FEEDING FILE

EXPRESSING MILK BY HAND

Advantages

● No special equipment is needed, only a wide-necked sterile container and clean hands

● Hand expressing mimics a baby's suckling action more closely than expressing by pump, so it may be a better way to maintain the milk supply

● Expressing by hand may be gentler than expressing with a pump.

Disadvantages

● It may take longer to express by hand than by pump

● Your hands may get tired.

How to hand express

● Use a hand to cup your breast from underneath, with your forefinger along the line where your areola (the dark area surrounding your nipple) and breast meet. Place your thumb on top of your breast, along the same line.

● Your milk is stored in reservoirs situated approximately below this line. These reservoirs need to be squeezed gently to extract the milk. You may need to move your hand slightly in towards your nipple or back towards your chest to find the milk reservoirs – experiment until you find the right place for you

● Gently squeeze your thumb and fingers together, pushing back and in towards your ribcage at the same time. This combined movement helps push the milk along the ducts towards the nipple, as well as squeezing it out

● Relax the pressure, then repeat the movement

● Your milk may take a minute or two to flow, so don't give up if nothing happens immediately

● Move your hand around your breast, so that you cover all the milk ducts. You could also change hands on the same breast

● If your hand gets tired, change sides, then come back to the first side later

● Sometimes it is easier to get the knack of hand expressing after you have been shown how. Your midwife, health visitor or breastfeeding counsellor should be able to help you

● The very best way to learn may be to watch someone who is able to do it – ask your breastfeeding counsellor if she knows someone who might show you how.

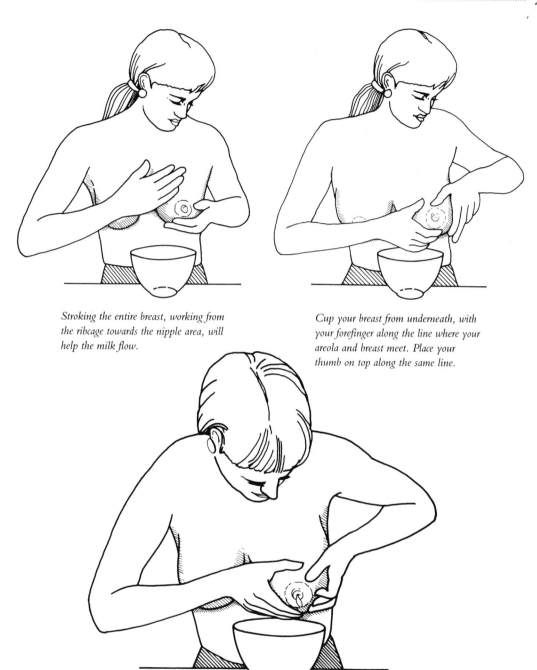

Stroking the entire breast, working from the ribcage towards the nipple area, will help the milk flow.

Cup your breast from underneath, with your forefinger along the line where your areola and breast meet. Place your thumb on top along the same line.

Gently squeeze your thumb and fingers together, pushing back and in towards your ribcage.

FEEDING FILE

TIPS FOR EXPRESSING MILK

● Expressing usually becomes easier and more productive with practice, so don't worry if you get only a little milk at first

● The best time to express varies from person to person. There may be a time when your breasts feel fuller, perhaps early morning. Once you return to work, a routine of expressing may be imposed by tea-breaks and hours of working

● When you are learning, try to choose a time when you are not rushed and won't be interrupted

● A warm, comfortable place with a comfortable chair is most conducive

● A relaxed atmosphere will help the milk to flow, so think about what helps you to relax: perhaps some music, or relaxation exercises beforehand

● Stroking the entire breast, working from the rib cage towards the nipple area will help to stimulate the milk to flow

● Warmth encourages the milk to flow, so try expressing after a bath or shower, or try putting a warm flannel on your breast, or hugging a hot water bottle

● Think about your baby, and your milk flowing. Sometimes it helps to have a photo of your baby nearby, or a tape of him

● Back massage may help the milk to flow. If there is someone who can do this, get him or her to stand behind you, with a fist either side of your spine, level with your breasts. Rub the fists up and down, gently but firmly

● Some mothers find that it is helpful to concentrate on other things to get their milk flowing: perhaps a TV programme, a book or some good conversation

● Try expressing from one breast while your baby is feeding from the other, or continue expressing just after a feed.

How much milk to express

● It can be difficult to know how much expressed milk your baby will need whilst you are away

● A rule of thumb used to work out roughly how much formula-fed babies drink is to allow 2½oz of milk for each pound of the baby's weight in 24 hours. So, for example, a 10lb baby might take 25oz of milk in 24 hours. This is a *very* rough guide: breastfed babies may take more or less than this, and their intake may not be evenly distributed throughout the day

● When you have been back at work for a week or two, you will have a better idea of how much milk your baby needs. Even so, an extra quantity in the fridge or freezer would be a useful 'back up' in case your baby's needs increase unexpectedly.

FEEDING FILE

STORING EXPRESSED BREAST MILK

● Use fresh, rather than frozen, breast milk whenever you can, as freezing has some effect on the nutrients and anti-infective properties of breast milk

● Expressed milk can be stored in a fridge for 24 hours or in a deep freeze for up to 3 months. You may read elsewhere that longer storage times are acceptable; we have used the most stringent recommendations here

● Store milk in the coldest part of the fridge, usually the back or bottom. It may be worth buying a fridge thermometer. Breast milk should be stored at 4°C or below

● After expressing, cool milk quickly in a container of cold water, then store it in the fridge, or in a well-insulated container with ice packs if you do not have access to a fridge at work. You can use the same container to transport fresh or frozen milk to your baby's carer

● To freeze milk, cool it quickly first, then freeze it in sterile plastic bags or lidded plastic containers, labelled and dated. Covered plastic ice-cube trays can be used for freezing, then cubes can be transferred to another container for storage

● Remember not to fill containers too full, to allow for expansion during freezing

● It can be useful to have milk frozen in small quantities so that you don't have to unfreeze, and perhaps waste, more milk than your baby needs

● Freshly expressed milk can be added to milk expressed or frozen earlier, but cool the new milk separately first, and don't add more than half the amount of milk already frozen to a pre-frozen batch

● Defrost frozen breast milk as quickly as possible, by holding the container under cool, then warmer running water, or by standing it in hot water. Use the same method for warming expressed milk, or use a bottle warmer

● Don't use a microwave to thaw or warm milk, as the milk may overheat, or heat unevenly, and some of the nutrients will be destroyed

● Thawed milk which has not been heated may be stored in the fridge for 24 hours, but any unused milk which has been warmed should be thrown out

● If the fat separates during storage, give the milk a good shake.

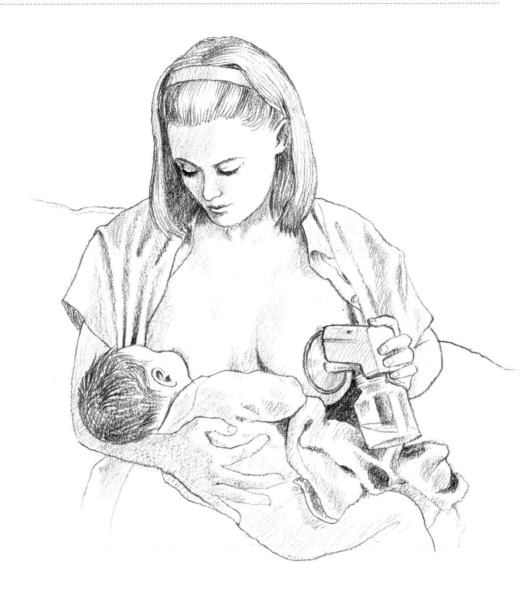

INTRODUCING CUPS OR BOTTLES

MANY BABIES adapt well to taking expressed breast milk, formula or other drinks by bottle or cup from their carer, and breastfeeding when you are there. A cup may be a good alternative to a bottle for babies who may become confused by the different sucking actions required for breast and bottle. Some breastfed babies are reluctant to take a bottle, and persistence may be needed. It can help to try different teats, or to warm the teat. Someone other than you – your baby associates you with breastfeeding – may be more successful in getting your baby to take a bottle.

About six weeks before going back to work, when her baby was about six months old, Natalie started to reduce the number of breast-feeds, so that her baby became accustomed to having fewer breast-feeds throughout the day: *'I tried replacing breastfeeds with various permutations of diluted fruit juice, water, formula milk, cow's milk and expressed breast milk, in cups with various types of spout, and bottles with various types of teat. This was to no avail as she never took a bottle success-fully and at this stage her cup skills were pretty basic. When we got down to three feeds a day I was reluctant to drop further feeds as I didn't feel she was drinking enough – staff at the nursery reported that she only took mouthfuls of fluids which I compared to the 8oz bottles of milk which her contemporaries were having. I was worried that she'd get dehydrated or constipated or start to wake up in the night demanding more feeds. I knew intellectually that she must be getting enough fluids, but I worried because she seemed to be drink-ing hardly anything.'*

Paula's daughter, Charlotte, would only accept breast milk from the breast: *'Once I was back at work it became apparent that Charlotte wasn't going to take breast milk from a bottle or a beaker or a spoon. Instead, the milk was used to mix up baby rice. The rice mixture was then stirred into fruit and vegetable purees.'*

Rita's baby was happy to take her milk from a bottle: *'I began to express milk fairly early on and once or twice each week my husband slept downstairs with the baby and gave him a bottle of my milk. It meant that I was able to get six or seven hours of unbroken sleep, and the baby had a bottle frequently enough to become used to it, but not so often as to break the routine of feed-ing from me.'*

THE NEED FOR SUPPORT

IN AN IDEAL world, all working mothers would have a longer period of paid maternity leave, with the option of flexible working hours or part-time work when they return. For breastfeeding mothers there would be a right to breastfeeding or expressing breaks during the working day, more childcare at the workplace or nearby, and comfortable, private facilities for expressing milk at work. At present, some mothers manage to negotiate reasonable arrangements for themselves and have good support from family, friends and employers.

Wendy's husband was her greatest support: *'On the whole, it has worked out fine, probably even better than if my husband had gone to work and I had stayed at home, because it is less tiring to go to work than to look after a baby and do the housework. What has made the whole experience relatively easy is the fact that my husband has been very supportive and really did everything at home. Also, we slept with the baby in our bed, which is good for the baby, good for me because I need to be with her, and good for my sleep too. Despite working full time, I am with my baby 16 hours a day with this arrangement.'*

Tessa returned to work as a full time ward sister working on a shift pattern when her baby was five months old: *'Baby fed at 5.30am – left for work at 6am having packed a supply of breast milk for Owen while at the nursery. My husband was a full-time student in his final year at university. He took Owen to the nursery in the morning and I collected him at 4.30pm when I finished my work. When I worked on a late shift until 9.30pm I took Owen to nursery and my husband collected him after his classes. When I collected him at 4.30pm I breastfed him again before taking him home as we live in a village 30 miles from the nursery – not a five-minute journey and he could not wait. When at home I then fed him on demand the rest of the evening and night. As he fed on one side I pumped and stored (either refrigerated or froze) the milk from the other side.*

Baby was up two-hourly to feed at night and wanted to suck all evening when we got home – all this on top of a day at work and shopping, housework etc. My husband was not really able to help with shopping and housework as he was at the time sitting his final exams. I had to be determined to make it succeed. Every time the baby fed at night it was not a case of a quick feed and down again. I had to force myself to get up, pump the milk from the other side, store it or freeze it, and re-sterilise all the pumping equipment for the next time. Having done all this I climbed back into bed.

I had desperately wanted to breastfeed to give my baby the best start in life and was determined to continue when I went back to work. He was a good feeder and that thankfully was not a problem. I loved breastfeeding and although it was tough at the time I consider it a great achievement on my behalf that my baby continued with breast milk while I worked full time.'

COMBINING BREASTFEEDING and work can be very demanding, particularly for mothers who work full time and whose babies are fully breastfed. Good support from others who have done or are doing it, co-operative employers, people who will help with practical tasks, and above all, people who think that it is worth all the effort, can make the task much easier.

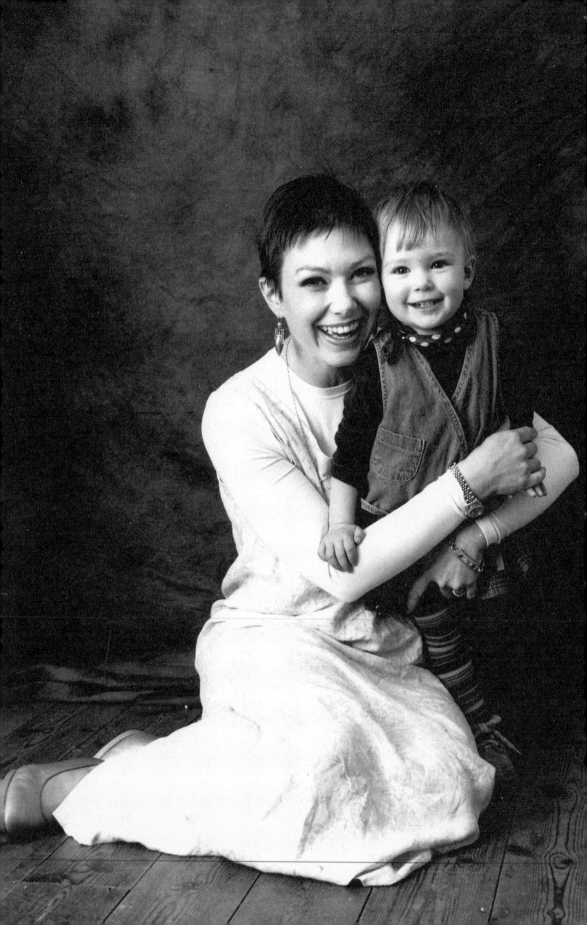

CHAPTER *__twelve__* *Finishing breastfeeding*

Finishing breastfeeding ends a very special relationship between a mother and her baby. You may finish almost as soon as you have started through experiencing too many difficulties or just deciding it is not for you. You may have breastfed for many months but reached the stage where your baby or you are ready to stop. For however long you breastfeed there is no doubt that it will have created a unique bond. The experience of breastfeeding may also have brought other rewards, such as a sense of fulfilment and achievement, and a boost to self-confidence. It is perhaps not surprising, then, that you may have mixed feelings when breastfeeding finishes and a new stage in your baby's life begins, as these three mothers did:

'My time as a breastfeeding mother is something I'll always remember with great pleasure. I was lucky to have few problems, although I found weaning quite difficult. The books say you drop one feed one week, substituting other food/drinks, then another, until the baby is weaned, but my daughter wasn't very interested in anything other than breastmilk. We managed it eventually but it was a struggle.'

'Part of me misses the special closeness of breastfeeding and the ability to comfort her instantly.'

'I was alarmed that two days after the last feed I just could not stop crying. A friend reassured me that "weaning grief" was a common experience and did not mean I was wrong to stop breastfeeding. I wish I had known about this in advance as I did not understand it and was afraid it was the onset of delayed postnatal depression. But the next day I felt normal again.'

Regrets may be stronger if your baby chooses to stop feeding before you had planned. Gemma enjoyed feeding Beth and remembers so

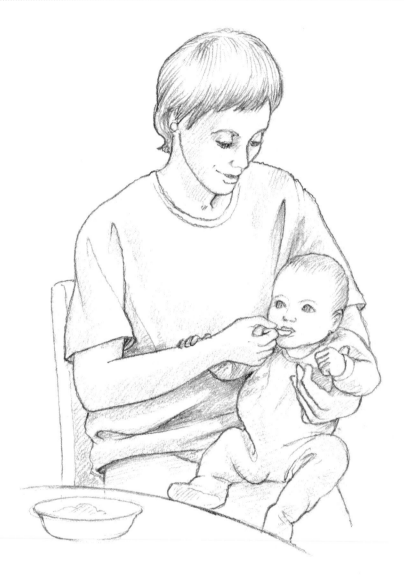

vividly the first feed she refused at about five or six months: *'It was at lunchtime and I felt rejected and sad, my little baby was becoming independent.'*

Joanna's first baby suddenly refused to feed when he was about nine months old: *'This was very traumatic emotionally as I had only heard and read about deciding when you wanted to stop feeding or trying to stop when the baby wanted to continue. It was also very much a physical problem for me as he was a baby who had been very reluctant to eat solid food and was still taking four or five large feeds a day from me.'*

YOU MAY be happy to stop breastfeeding. You may have fed for as long as you intended, and be ready to move on to a different relationship with your baby.

Jane's baby is now nine months: *'Over the last three weeks or so I've cut down on breastfeeding so that she usually just has a feed at bedtime – 7pm. I'm happy with this and actually quite looking forward to stopping – a feeling I'm surprised at. I thought I'd be reluctant to stop feeding our last baby.'*

SOMETIMES IT may be a relief to stop breastfeeding, especially if the experience has not been a positive one.

Kate was advised by her health visitor to stop breastfeeding and change to formula feeds: *'Well, it would be wrong to say that everything was rosy from that day onwards, but I can honestly say that things did improve. I no longer had this baby sucking at me continuously and I managed to sleep for a number of hours at a time rather than minutes. I am quite sure that if I had continued the breastfeeding battle it would have taken considerably longer for my daughter and me to develop the fantastic relationship we now have, if at all.'*

WHO CHOOSES WHEN TO STOP?

THE BEST time to start weaning your baby from the breast depends on your feelings and your individual breastfeeding circumstances. Sometimes your baby leads the way with weaning, gradually losing interest in breastfeeding as he grows older and is distracted by new interests.

Gill found weaning a fairly natural process: *'After five months I found that his attention was moving to the outside world and he constantly moved off the breast at the slightest distraction, so I breastfed him at quiet times (morning, evening and in the night if necessary) but gave him a bottle during the day when distractions prevailed. By seven months he was beginning to lose interest and dropped the evening feed and finally at eight months he no longer wanted the breast at all. I was very pleased that he had chosen when to stop feeding from me, although I accept that he may have done this more quickly as a result of having sampled the alternative of the bottle.'*

Anna's daughter waited a bit longer before making her feelings clear: *'When she was 14 months old, she sat on my lap one bedtime and said "juice". I obeyed this most definite command; she settled. The following evening I offered my slightly over-full breast and she obligingly had a last feed. We both seemed to know it was a savoured closeness.'*

YOU MAY decide yourself when to begin weaning your baby from the breast, either because you have fed for as long as you want to, or for other reasons, such as returning to work or wanting to become pregnant. Sometimes you may be influenced by comments from friends or relatives.

These influences can be positive, as they were for Jean: *'I started to wean Roberta at four months. One new friend was breastfeeding her second child, the*

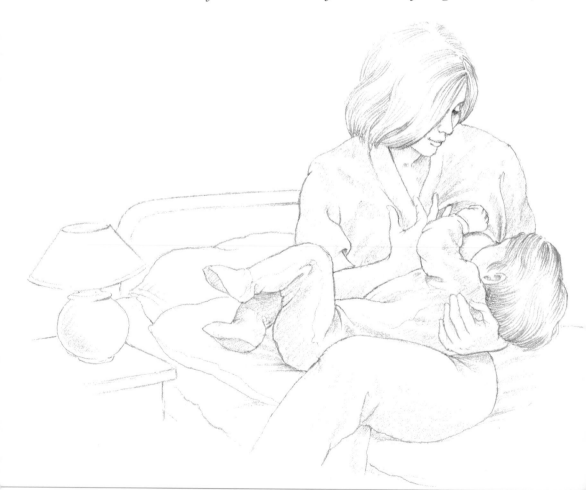

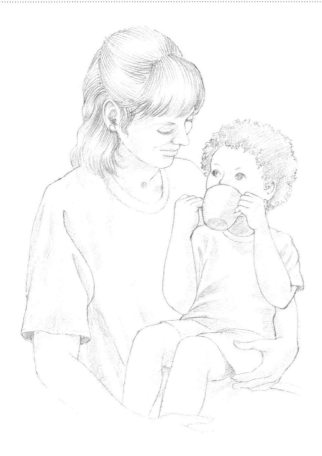

same age as Roberta, and the fact that she was still happily feeding at six months gave me comfort against comments such as "you're still feeding then?" '

Anne-Marie's family influences were less positive: *'My mother and sister felt that I was too fanatical about breastfeeding and why was I putting myself and my baby through all this anguish. My mum fed me for six weeks and then she didn't have enough milk. So she couldn't understand why I was so against formula. My sister had topped up and eventually gone over to bottle-feeding with her two children. The pressure was subtle, I doubt they know how upsetting it was, but I got their "message" loud and clear.'*

It is valuable to share how you feel about stopping breastfeeding with your partner. Kirsty and her husband saw the breastfeeding relationship differently: *'Together, my husband Sandy and I decided that I should stop breastfeeding during our summer holiday which would be when Jim was*

17 months old. Sandy saw Jim's breastfeeding as a habit to be broken. I saw it as an integral part of our relationship, as intimate as it was fulfilling for both of us. Consequently, when I stopped feeding both my mind and body ached to feed Jim again, whereas with each opportunity for a feed refused, Sandy felt that I was one step nearer my goal. Having a different idea of breastfeeding from my husband and not talking about this openly and early enough was one of the things which made stopping more traumatic than it might otherwise have been.'

Angela's daughter, Carol, was weaned from the breast on the advice of her GP: *'I didn't want to stop breastfeeding, but I was deeply depressed, and my doctor advised me to wean her for the sake of my health, and I reluctantly agreed that it might help. I don't remember it upsetting her as much as I had expected, but I decided to give her a bottle in the evenings, as she'd always been a "sucky" baby, but had never sucked her thumb, and it seemed a bit hard to suddenly deprive her of her comfort habit.'*

SOME BABIES are comfortable with replacing breastfeeds with other drinks or food, or do not object to being diverted from breastfeeding.

Ruth started to wean Lily gradually at about five months. She took solids very well. As she had more solids, she gradually reduced her breastfeeds: *'I cut out the morning feed first, decreasing the sucking time by one minute at a time. Once the morning feed was cut out, I went on to cut out the night feed. Although it was my decision to stop the breastfeeding completely, I did miss the closeness and warmth of feeding my baby. For a few weeks it was as though Lily didn't need me any more. She didn't bat an eyelid at not being breastfed. I am grateful, though, that it was a gradual process and not at all traumatic.'*

SOME BABIES are reluctant to be weaned from the breast. Sometimes older babies and toddlers become dedicated and determined breastfeeders and you and your partner may need to devise strategies to help your child accept the end of breastfeeding. Substitutes will be needed for the comfort and security which your baby or child has gained from breastfeeding, as well as for the breast milk itself.

Christine and her husband worked together to encourage their son to alter his pattern: *'When I finally decided it was time to start weaning my*

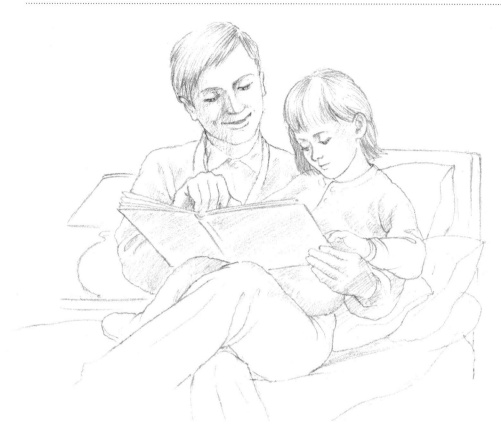

son from the breast, he had other ideas. He was by that stage eating and drinking plenty of other things, but breastfeeding was still important to him – in the morning, at nap time and at bedtime. My husband put him to bed for a week whilst I made myself scarce, which ended the bedtime feed. At nap time I took to pushing him in the buggy, rather than sitting down on the sofa with him as I had done previously. The morning feed was most difficult as it usually took place at about 5.30am and allowed us all some extra rest. I was very reluctant to make myself unavailable by getting up, so this feed carried on until I got pregnant again, at which point we started putting Chris to bed later and he gradually woke later in the morning so that I could face getting up and offering breakfast rather than a feed.'

Bedtime was the most difficult time for Polly: *'As John grew older, he was persuaded to drink juice during the day, but I couldn't work out how to put a baby to bed without a feed, as he still fell asleep at the breast. I needed the morning feed to remove the milk manufactured during the night. By the time he was 16 months old, we had been down to two feeds a day for months, but were no nearer dropping them. Nick had always bathed John, we dried and dressed him between us, then I fed him prior to going to bed. We finally agreed that for the next week, I would hide during the bath, and Nick would put him to bed. This worked in just a week. It took rather longer for the milk supply to completely dry up, and I lived on painkillers for about three days. So much for the people who said John couldn't possibly be taking much milk at his age, and was just comfort-sucking.'*

STOPPING BECAUSE OF DIFFICULTIES

AT PRESENT, many women who stop breastfeeding do so not because they feel ready to wean the baby, but because they are experiencing breastfeeding difficulties which seem not to be easily resolved. Unfortunately, for some women, the pain (both physical and emotional) associated with breastfeeding is just too much to bear and they decide, often with mixed feelings, to add formula feeds to breastfeeding. Introducing formula under these circumstances may lead to the end of breastfeeding completely, as these mothers discovered:

'By the end of the second week the cracked nipple had not healed and was bleeding when feeding on it or using the breast pump on it. I would have persevered but my baby was unsettled and obviously very hungry. This was the crucial time when I made the decision to give him a bottle. He turned into a different baby, obviously satisfied and much more content. I was bitterly disappointed at what I saw as my failure to breastfeed but felt that he would be a happier baby if I topped him up with bottles. I gradually increased bottles and decreased breast until I stopped breastfeeding completely when my son was six weeks old.'

'After a really grim evening when the baby had been trying to feed for about five hours, my husband made the decision for me that we had to bottle-feed. I couldn't have made the decision for myself – I would have felt too guilty. By then the baby was ten days old and had not had one proper breastfeed. He took the formula rapturously, and hasn't looked back since. I expressed milk as much as I could but after only three weeks it dried up, which really disappointed me.'

IF YOU have stopped breastfeeding because of difficulties, you may be left with very strong feelings – of disappointment, failure, guilt, anger or sadness.

Stopping breastfeeding was an emotional time for Celia: '*After four and a half weeks I finally gave in and reverted to bottle-feeding feeling totally depressed and a complete failure as a mum. I felt very sad that no one seemed to have any advice that could have helped me over those first difficult weeks. My sense of failure was great and the guilt that I had given in where others seemed to have persevered is still with me now. I was very envious of all breast-feeding mums. I also feel that had I had access to greater support in the form of other mums who were breastfeeding or had breastfed, I would have been encouraged to continue.*'

Stopping breastfeeding seemed rational to Debbie, but emotionally she was less sure: '*Bottles allowed me independence, stretches of time when I could actually feed myself and think about other things. Up until that point I had rarely left the baby apart from going to the toilet. Life became easier, apart from the necessary preparation of formula milk, but my guilt and feelings of failure are still with me. I did not feel any sense of love for my baby when she was born. I was very anxious that she should not have anything wrong. Afterwards I felt quite sick with responsibility. Through breastfeeding I was able to bond with my daughter and grow to love her. Now, when I am unable to feed her myself and see her hands on the bottle I am upset because I wish they were holding on to me.*'

Connie's decision was precipitated by illness, but it was no less hard for her: '*Unfortunately at four months I contracted a stomach virus and was readmitted to hospital with dehydration. I then decided to stop breastfeeding. I was exhausted. I expressed the milk for a few days until I had made my decision. This also eased the pain and leakage from engorged breasts. This was a very sad time for me. Not only did I miss my baby, I felt I had failed again. We live at the other end of the country to our families so there was no one to help or put things in perspective then.*'

IT SEEMS as though these women felt that their inability to succeed with breastfeeding was a failure: something they were, at least in part, responsible for. These are common feelings. You may accept them and go on to hope you might be able to 'get it right' next time. You may feel guilty. If you choose to breastfeed and are not enabled to, then yes, there has been a failure; but does it mean you have failed? Surely not.

You need help and support to succeed. If the help and support is not available or is not skilled, and you do not succeed with breast-feeding, could the fault lie with the system of support? These mothers think so.

Shirley's main feeling is one of anger that the help available was so inadequate: '*Having talked to other mothers, I know now that my problem was not uncommon and with proper advice could have been resolved. Everyone placed such emphasis on breastfeeding antenatally but when the time came no one seemed to have the skills needed to make it work. I began to wonder if they'd received any training in breastfeeding.*'

Sandra feels bitter that she didn't have the support she needed when trying to breastfeed her first two children: '*It seems to me that too many of the health professionals that I met were too ready to advise the bottle at the first sign of any problems, rather than giving realistic support to enable me to succeed at feeding. In other words all the advice that seemed to be available is geared around giving up a supposedly futile attempt – with platitudes such as .... "formula is so good nowadays that when she is a year old you won't be able to tell whether she was breast or bottle-fed". I allowed myself to believe this the first time but now I know I can breastfeed successfully I feel cheated.*'

Amanda assumed her new baby would be bottle-fed as she had been unable to breastfeed her first baby, Jo, but: '*As time went on I began to find out more about how to make breastfeeding successful, and to my horror I discovered that my inability to feed Jo had been due to our experiences in hospital. My biggest mistake, I believe, was that I assumed that the hospital staff knew enough and cared enough about breastfeeding to give me the information and support I needed.*'

AN UNSUCCESSFUL breastfeeding experience can be a major source of distress. In this situation, you may find it helpful to contact a breast-feeding counsellor to talk over what has happened. It is important to remember that however long or short your breastfeeding experience, you gave your child the best start in life.

FEEDING FILE

WEANING YOUR BABY FROM THE BREAST

When to wean

● There is no right age or stage at which to begin weaning or to stop breastfeeding altogether. The decision depends on the feelings and circumstances of each individual breastfeeding pair

● If you can, try to avoid starting at times which are likely to be stressful for you or your baby, for example when you return to work or when she is teething

● It may help to discuss your plans for weaning, and your feelings about it, with a health visitor or breastfeeding counsellor.

What should substitute for breast milk?

● This will depend on the age and preferences of your baby. Milk is an important source of nutrition throughout your baby's first two years

● If you stop breastfeeding before your baby is a year old, he will probably need some formula milk. Ordinary cow's milk is not recommended for drinks until babies are a year old, although whole cow's milk is suitable for use in cooking and with cereal

● If your baby is eating solids and still having some breastfeeds, you could satisfy his thirst at other times with cooled, boiled water or well-diluted fruit juice

● Many experts feel that 'follow-on milks', advertised for babies of six months and over, have no real advantage over other types of formula and are more expensive.[62]

Starting to wean

● If there is a time of day when your baby is less interested in breastfeeding, start by cutting down or dropping that feed: perhaps at lunch time, when he has had something else to eat

● Avoid starting with a feed which is very important as a source of comfort for your baby, such as his bedtime feed

● If your baby is reluctant to take formula milk in a bottle from you, someone else may have more success – she associates you with breastfeeding. You can also try different teats, or softening the teat in boiled water

● Unless you need to wean your baby rapidly, allow several days or weeks between each feed you drop. This will allow both of you time to adjust.

FEEDING FILE

Replacing the emotional benefits of breastfeeding

● You may need to help your baby find substitutes for the feelings of comfort, security and closeness which he gets from breastfeeding. Some things which may help are:
    a soft toy, special piece of clothing or blanket which he can cuddle;
    extra cuddles and stroking from you and others whom he loves;
    at bedtime, a lullaby or a story instead of a feed.

Bottles or cups?

● The choice of a bottle, a beaker with a spout or a cup for your baby depends on his age and preferences
● If he is being weaned from the breast completely, or he is only a few months old, he may want the comfort and familiarity of sucking from a bottle

● If she is older and will be partially breastfeeding for a time she may be happy to take her other drinks from a beaker or a cup
● Some babies become proficient at drinking from a small beaker or cup from about three or four months, which may be helpful if they refuse a bottle.

Babies who don't want to stop breastfeeding

● Some babies choose to stop feeding themselves but others are extremely reluctant to stop, particularly older babies and toddlers who feed often
● You may need to devise strategies to help your baby stop feeding with the minimum of distress
● If possible, try to start at a time when there will be extra help or diversions available, for example in summer when your child can play outside, or when your partner or other supportive person can be around
● Think about the times at which your child usually wants to feed and alter your routine, so that familiar prompts and situations for breastfeeding are removed. For example, if you normally sit together on the sofa for a feed before his nap, go out with the pushchair instead

● If it is difficult to cut out feeds, start by reducing their length
● In the morning, get up for an early breakfast instead of giving a feed, if you or your partner can bear it
● At night, your partner or someone else who is close to your child could put him to bed whilst you go out
● The most difficult time may be during the night, when there are no other distractions and everyone needs to sleep. You might decide that your partner or another adult whom your child knows well will go to your child and comfort him for as long as necessary
● Some mothers go away for the night or weekend when ending night feeds. Leaving your child to cry, but going regularly to reassure him, is a stressful strategy for all concerned but might be considered if all else fails.

FEEDING FILE

Weaning and you

● If possible, gradual weaning is preferable, that is cutting out a feed every few days or weeks, or less frequently. This will give your body time to adjust to producing less milk, minimising the possibility of overfull and sore breasts

● Gradual weaning allows a slower decline in the level of the hormone prolactin which is produced during breastfeeding. A sudden drop in prolactin levels can sometimes lead to feelings of depression

● If your breasts become full and hard at any stage during weaning, because you are producing more milk than your baby now needs, it may help to:

● Take a hot bath or shower, or use warm flannels on your breasts to encourage a small amount of milk to leak from the breasts

● Express just enough milk to relieve the fullness in your breasts until you start to produce less milk

● Very gently massage your breasts towards the nipples to keep them free of lumps

● Use cold compresses or cabbage leaves inside your bra to relieve soreness and reduce swelling

● Take painkillers (not aspirin)

● Use any of the suggestions in Chapter Four for relieving breast fullness.

Where to get help with weaning

People to talk to:
● Your health visitor
● An NCT breastfeeding counsellor
● A La Leche League leader
● Other mothers who have breastfed and weaned their babies.

Suggested reading:
● *Feeding your child from birth to three*, by Heather Welford. Health Education Authority, 1994.

THE FUTURE

IN RECOGNITION of the need to provide a better service for breast-feeding mothers, several government initiatives have been established to improve the care of and support for breastfeeding mothers and to further public education about the value of breastfeeding. Training for health professionals, preparing or updating local breastfeeding policies, raising public awareness of breastfeeding, research, and preparing good information on breastfeeding for mothers; all these exciting initiatives are happening in Britain today. The future looks brighter for breastfeeding. These three mothers have the last word:

'I very much enjoyed breastfeeding my two daughters and want to tell other mothers about this feeling of satisfaction and pleasure. To me, there is no greater bond between mother and child, no more pleasurable feeling than feeding your own baby, being able to comfort her with the breast immediately and

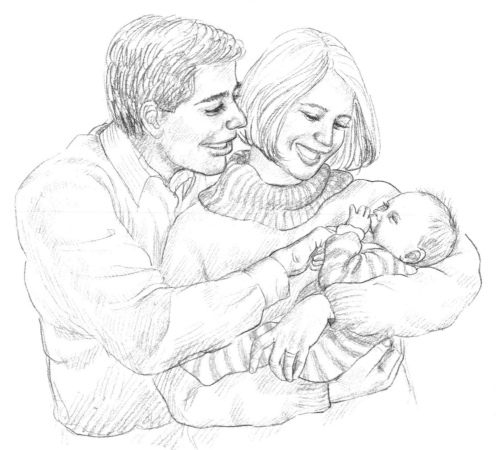

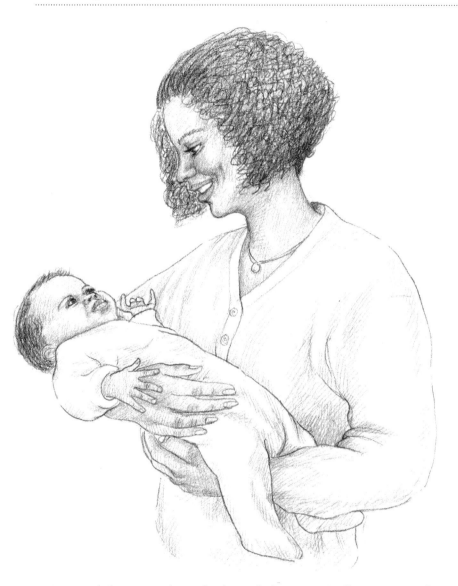

seeing your baby growing bigger by the week, knowing it's all your own work!'
'Breastfeeding my children from almost helpless, unfocused infants, through to
demonstrative little people who show their obvious enjoyment and preference
for the gorgeous, sweet milk which they consider their right was a fantastic
experience.'

'My breastfeeding experience has been one of the most rewarding things in my
life. To know that I gave my three children the best start they could have and to
have enjoyed it so much myself is paramount to my feelings about motherhood.'

Further reading

Chloe Fisher, Mary Renfrew and Suzanne Arms. *Bestfeeding*. Celestial Arts.

Breastfeeding Twins, Triplets or More. Twins & Multiple Births Association (leaflet).

Gabrielle Palmer. *The Politics of Breastfeeding*. Pandora. 2nd ed.

The Art of Breastfeeding. La Leche League.

Mary Smale. *The National Childbirth Trust Book of Breastfeeding*. Vermilion.

NCT publications

The NCT produces leaflets and booklets on many aspects of birth and parenthood, including breastfeeding. A catalogue of the current titles is available by post from: NCT (Maternity Sales) Ltd., Burnfield Avenue, Glasgow G46 7TL. Tel. 0141 633 5552. (Also available on tape via RNIB Redhill, Philanthropic Road, Redhill, Surrey RH1 4DG. Tel. 01737 768935.)

Video

Breast Is Best: about mother's milk, breastfeeding and early contact with the newborn. 35 mins. Directed by Gro Nylander, co-ordinator of the Baby Friendly Hospital Initiative in Norway. Available from Baby Milk Action.

Where to get help

Organisations which offer help with breastfeeding and counselling:

National Childbirth Trust,

Alexandra House,
Oldham Terrace,
Acton,
London W3 6NH.
Tel. 0181 992 8637

Breastfeeding counsellors are available to all mothers. Telephone for details of your nearest counsellor. NCT breastfeeding counsellors are ready to listen to any mother who wishes to contact them and to see her problems, large or small, from a mother's point of view. They encourage mothers to talk freely about their feeding experiences and treat such discussions as strictly confidential. They try to be sensitive to the mothers' needs and to understand what may not always be explicitly stated. NCT breastfeeding counsellors aim to give sound factual information and can usually offer practical help, for example when a breast pump is needed. Their aim is not, however, to advocate a particular solution but to bolster a breastfeeding woman's confidence in her ability to cope and to encourage her to make her own decisions. Counsellors are trained to be flexible in their attitudes to infant feeding and to be positive and supportive to all mothers whether they choose to breastfeed or decide ultimately to bottle-feed.

La Leche League

BM 3424
London WC1N 3XX
Tel. 0171 242 1278

Counsellors available to all mothers who are breastfeeding. Telephone for details of your nearest group.

Association of Breastfeeding Mothers

26 Holmeshaw Close
London SE26 4TH
Tel. 0181 778 4769

Offers support for breastfeeding mothers.

Organisations which offer a counselling service:

British Association of Counselling
1 Regent Place, Rugby
Warwickshire CV21 2PJ

Other organisations:

Baby Milk Action

23 St. Andrew's Street
Cambridge CB2 3AX
Tel. 01223 464420

A non-profit organisation which aims to halt the commercial promotion of bottle-feeding and to protect and promote good infant nutrition. Promotes Nestlé boycott in UK.

References

1. White, A, Freeth, S and O'Brien, M 1992: *Infant Feeding 1990*. HMSO. (A survey carried out by the Social Survey Division of the Office of Population Censuses and Surveys, SS1299.)

2. Littman, H, Medendorp, S V & Goldfarb, J 1994: The decision to breastfeed: the importance of fathers' approval. *Clinical Pediatrics*, vol. 33, no. 4, pp214–219.

3. MAIN Trial Collaborative Group 1994: Preparing for breastfeeding: treatment of inverted and non-protractile nipples in pregnancy. *Midwifery*, vol. 10, pp200–214.

4. Heinig, M J, Nommsen, L A & Dewey, K G 1992: Lactation and postpartum weight loss. *Mechanisms Regulating Lactation and Infant Nutrition Utilization*, vol. 30, pp397–400.

5. Dewey, K G, Heinig, M J & Nommsen, L A 1993: Maternal weight loss patterns during prolonged lactation. *Am. J. Clin. Nutr.*, vol. 58, pp162–166.

6. Newcomb, B E *et al* 1994: Lactation and a reduced risk of premenopausal breast cancer. *New Engl. J. Med.*, vol. 330, no. 2, pp81–87.

7. UK National Case-Control Study Group 1993: Breastfeeding and risk of breast cancer in young women. *Br. Med. J.*, vol. 307, no. 6895, pp17–20.

8. Cancer and Steroid Hormone Study, CDC/NICHHD 1987: The reduction in risk of ovarian cancer associated with oral contraceptive use. *New Engl. J. Med.*, vol. 316, pp650–655.

9. Singh, K K, Suchindran, C M & Singh, K 1993: Effects of breastfeeding after resumption of menstruation on waiting time to next conception. *Human Biol.*, vol. 65, pp71–86.

10. Kennedy, K I & Visness, C M 1992: Contraceptive efficacy of lactational amenorrhoea. *Lancet*, vol. 339, pp227–230.

11. Sowers, M *et al* 1993: Changes in bone density with lactation. *J. Am. Med. Assoc.*, vol. 269, pp3130–3135.

12. Cummings, R G & Klineberg, R J 1993: Breastfeeding and other reproductive factors and the risk of hip fracture in elderly women. *Int. J. Epidemiol.*, vol. 2, no. 4, pp684–691.

13. Cockburn, F *et al* 1995: Effect of diet on the fatty acid composition of the major phospholipids of infant cerebral cortex. *Arch. Dis. Childh.*, vol. 72, pp198–203.

14. Makrides, M *et al* 1995: Are long-chain polyunsaturated fatty acids essential nutrients in infancy? *Lancet*, vol. 345, pp1463–1468.

15. Goldman, A S 1993: The immune system of human milk: antimicrobial, anti-inflammatory and immunomodulating properties. *Pediatr. Infect. Dis. J.*, vol. 12, pp664–671.

16. Rogan, W G & Gladen, B C 1993: Breastfeeding and cognitive development. *Early Human Devel.*, vol. 31, pp181–193.

17. Lanting, C I *et al* 1994: Neurological differences between nine-year-old children fed breast milk or formula milk as babies. *Lancet*, vol. 344, pp1319–1322.

18. Lucas, A *et al* 1992: Breast milk and subsequent intelligence quotient in children born preterm. *Lancet*, vol. 339, pp261–264.

19. Lucas, A *et al* 1994: A randomised multicentre study of human milk versus formula and later development in preterm infants. *Arch. Dis. Childh.*, vol. 70, no. 2, ppF141–F146.

20. Birch, E *et al* 1993: Breastfeeding and

optimal visual development. *J. Pediatr. Opthalmol. Strabismus*, vol. 30, pp33–38.

21. Howie, P W *et al* 1990: Protective effect of breastfeeding against infection. *Br. Med. J.*, vol. 300, no. 6716, pp11–16.

22. Brock, J 1993: Breastfeeding – the immunological case. *New Generation Digest*, no. 4, pp5–6.

23. Lucas, A & Cole, T J 1990: Breast milk and neonatal necrotising enterocolitis. *Lancet*, vol. 336, pp1519–1523.

24. Burr, M L *et al* 1993: Infant feeding, wheezing and allergy: a prospective study. *Arch. Dis. Childh.*, vol. 68, pp724–728.

25. Wright, L *et al* 1989: Breastfeeding and lower respiratory tract illness in the first year of life. *Br. Med. J.*, vol. 299, pp946–949.

26. Duncan, B *et al* 1993: Exclusive breastfeeding for at least four months protects against otitis media. *Pediatrics*, vol. 91, no. 5, pp867–872.

27. Aniansson, G *et al* 1994: A prospective cohort study on breastfeeding and otitis media in Swedish infants. *Pediatr. Infect. Dis. J.*, vol. 13, pp183–188.

28. Karajalainen, J *et al* 1992: A bovine albumin peptide as a possible trigger of insulin-dependent diabetes. *New Engl. J. Med.*, vol. 327, pp302–307.

29. Virtanen, S M *et al* 1993: Early introduction of dairy products associated with increased risk of IDDM in Finnish children. *Diabetes*, vol. 42, pp1786–1790.

30. Monte, W C, Johnston, C S & Roll, L E 1994: Bovine serum albumin detected in infant formula is a possible trigger for insulin-dependent diabetes mellitus. *J. Amer. Diet. Assoc.*, vol. 94, pp314–316.

31. Businco, L & Cantani, A 1990: Prevention of childhood allergy by dietary manipulation. *Clin. Exper. Allergy*, vol. 20, suppl. 3, pp9–14.

32. Mepham, B 1991: Suckling-induced stimulation of breast milk. *New Generation*, vol. 10, no. 2, pp31–32.

33. Inch, S and Garforth, S: Establishing and maintaining breastfeeding. In: Chalmers, M, Enkin, M and Keirse, M (eds) 1989: *Effective care in pregnancy and childbirth*. Oxford Univ Pr. pp1364.

34. Royal College of Midwives 1991: *Successful breastfeeding: a practical guide for midwives and others supporting breastfeeding mothers*. Churchill Livingstone. pp27–29.

35. Hey, E 1995: Neonatal jaundice – how much do we really know? *MIDIRS Midwifery Digest*, vol. 5, no. 1, pp4–8.

36. De Carvalho, M 1981: Effects of water supplementation on physiological jaundice in breastfed babies. *Arch. Dis. Childhood*, vol. 56, no. 7, pp568–569.

37. Beeken, S & Waterston, T 1992: Health service support of breastfeeding – are we practising what we preach? *Br. Med. J.*, vol. 305, pp285–287.

38. Welford, H 1995: Bournemouth put breastfeeding first. *Modern Midwife*, vol. 5, no. 6, pp5–6.

39. Hawdon, J M, Ward Platt, M P and Aynsley Green, A 1992: Neonatal hypoglycaemia – blood glucose monitoring and baby feeding. *Midwifery*, vol. 9, pp3–6.

40. Glasier, A S, McNeilly, A S and Howie, P W 1984: The prolactin response to suckling. *Clinical Endocrinology*, vol. 21, pp109–116.

41. Director General of WHO 1992: Report, EB93/17. WHO, Geneva.

42. From *Protecting, Promoting and Supporting Breastfeeding: the special role of maternity services – a joint WHO/UNICEF statement*. 1989.

43. Glazener, C *et al* Health Services Research Unit, University of Aberdeen. Main research findings forthcoming, empirical evidence submitted to the House of Commons Health Committee, January 1992. Published in the *Second Report from the Health Committee: Maternity Services (Winterton Report) 1992*. vol. 1. House of Commons Session 1991–92.

44. Whitehead, R G and Paul, A A 1984: Growth charts and the assessment of infant

feeding practices in the western world and in developing countries. *Early Human Development*, vol. 9, pp187–207.

45. Dewey, K G *et al* 1992: Growth of breast-fed and formula fed infants from 0–18 months: the Darling (Davis Area Research on Lactation, Infant Nutrition and Growth) study. *Pediatrics*, vol. 89, pp1035–1041.

46. Gribble, Ginny 1995: A mother's manifesto. *New Generation*, vol. 14, no. 2, pp14–15.

47. See, for example, Redbridge Health Authority 1990: *Policy Statement on Breastfeeding in Public Areas of Health Authority Premises*.

48. Forsyth, J S *et al* 1993: Relation between early introduction of solid food to infants and their weight and illnesses during the first two years of life. *British Medical Journal*, vol. 306, pp1572–1576.

49. Fildes, V 1988: *Wet nursing: a history from antiquity to the present*. Blackwell.

50. Tyson, J E 1977: *Nursing and prolactin secretion*. Academic Press.

51. Woolridge, M W *et al* 1980: Effect of a traditional and of a new nipple shield on sucking patterns and milk flow. *Early Human Development*, vol. 4, pp357–362.

52. Auerback, K G 1990: The effect of nipple shields on maternal milk volume. *Journal of Obstetric and Neonatal Nursing*, vol. 19, no. 5, pp419–427.

53. Jakobsson, I and Lindberg, T 1983: Cow's milk proteins cause infantile colic in breastfed infants: a double-blind crossover study. *Paediatrics*, vol. 71, pp268–271.

54. Woolridge, M and Fisher, C 1988: Colic, 'overfeeding', and symptoms of lactose malabsorption in the breastfed baby: a possible artifact of feed management? *Lancet*, no. 8605, pp382–384.

55. Williams, A F 1993: Human milk and the preterm baby. *British Medical Journal*, vol. 306, pp1628–1629.

56. Williams, A F 1994: Is breastfeeding beneficial in the UK? Statement of the Standing Committee on Nutrition of the British Paediatric Association. *Arch. Dis. Childh.*, vol. 71, pp376–380.

57. Howie, P *et al* 1980: The relationship between suckling induced prolactin metabolism. *J. Clin. Endocrinol Metab.*, vol. 50, pp670–673.

58. Howie, P 1985: Breastfeeding – a new understanding. *Midwives Chronicle*, July, pp184–192.

59. Jones, E 1994: Breastfeeding in the preterm infant. *Modern Midwife*, vol. 4, no. 1, pp22–26.

60. DeCarvalho, M *et al* 1985: frequency of milk expression and milk production by mothers of non-nursing premature neonates. AJDC, vol. 139, pp483–485.

61. Minchin, M 1987: Premature babies: why breast is best. *New Generation*, vol. 6, no. 3, pp36–37.

62. Palmer, G 1993: Any old iron? *Health Visitor*, vol. 66, no. 7, pp248–249, 252.

Index